Alcohol dependence and smoking behaviour

Edited by
GRIFFITH EDWARDS
M. A. H. RUSSELL
DAVID HAWKS
MAXINE MacCAFFERTY
on behalf of
The Addiction Research Unit,
Institute of Psychiatry,
University of London

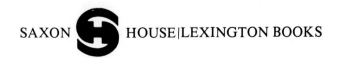
SAXON HOUSE|LEXINGTON BOOKS

Published by
SAXON HOUSE, D. C. Heath Ltd.
Westmead, Farnborough, Hants., England.

Jointly with
LEXINGTON BOOKS, D. C. Heath & Co.
Lexington, Mass. USA.

ISBN 0 347 01127 6
Library of Congress Catalog Card Number 75-30137
Printed in Great Britain by Butler and Tanner, Frome and London.

Contents

Acknowledgements

The acknowledgements section which is a common feature of any book of this type, often seems only a rather formal listing – the due and necessary mention of the wig maker, hosier, and cigarette manufacturer on the theatre programme. In this particular instance we would wish to state very clearly that our thanks are more than formal. The Addiction Research Unit owes immense gratitude to a wide range of people, who have together made it possible to put on the play. In preparing this list of acknowledgements we were again made aware of the extraordinary co-operative phenomenon of which this sort of research constitutes – the varieties of trust, co-operation, generosities, friendships, technical skills, that together make possible the play.

The listing is incomplete, and the order is rather arbitrary. We would though wish to start by thanking Sir Denis Hill, who as Head of the Department of Psychiatry of the Institute of Psychiatry has given the Unit absolutely crucial support. Early encouragement also came from the late Sir Aubrey Lewis. The role of Dr D. L. Davies in aiding the setting up of initial alcoholism studies deserves special mention. Dr Philip Connell (Director of the Bethlem–Maudsley Drug Dependence Clinical Research and Treatment Unit) has been a constant source of wise and generous counsel. The contribution of Dr A. N. Oppenheim (Reader in Social Psychology, London School of Economics) to the building of an inter-disciplinary Unit has been in many ways indispensable. Since the Unit received a consolidated DHSS/MRC programme grant useful guidance has been given by an Advisory Committee under the Chairmanship of Sir Martin Roth: we would thank Sir Martin and his colleagues not only in their formal role but also for tangible friendship.

The major financial support for the research has come in turn from the Bethlem–Maudsley Research Fund, the Nuffield Foundation, and currently from the Medical Research Council and the Department of Health and Social Security. To these funding bodies who have so generously financed studies on often very sensitive questions, while allowing the research team autonomy of judgement, special gratitude is owed. We also gratefully acknowledge smaller grants from, respectively, the Helping Hand Organisation and the Joint Research Board of St. Bartholomew's Hospital for help with two particular studies.

We acknowledge with gratitude advice and assistance given us by Dr H. David Archibald, Dr Michael Ashley-Miller, Dr A. A. Baker, Dr Keith Ball,

Dr D. H. Beese, Dr Douglas Bennett, Dr J. L. T. Birley, Dr E. R. Bransby, Dr Monamy Buckle, Dr Denis Cahal, Mr D. Cordy, Dr T. A. Dibly, Dr Joan Faulkner, Dr S. L. Gauntlett, Dr M. M. Glatt, Dr Roy Goulding, Dr Malcolm Lader, Dr Isaac Marks, Dr Alan Mawson, Miss Joy Mott, Professor M. H. Peston, Professor Michael Shepherd, Dr Alan Sippert, Professor Hannah Steinberg, Mr G. F. Todd, Professor Nigel Walker, and Professor John Wing. We have in various studies relied on use of DHSS and Home Office records, and we would particularly acknowledge the protection of subject anonymity which has been afforded. The assistance of the Central Statistical Officer, HM Customs and Excise, the Home Office Research Unit and the Tobacco Research Council is gratefully noted.

For access to research populations we have to thank many persons and organisations. We are indebted to staff at chest clinics who have referred patients for smoking studies, and in particular to Dr W. L. Ashton, Dr B. J. Malley, Mr W. E. D. Moore, Mr K. Robertson and Dr H. O. Williams. Generous co-operation in mounting a variety of surveys has been given by magistrates and court officials, prison authorities and staff, probation officers, college authorities, student unions, medical committees and governing bodies of hospitals, the staff of Camberwell Reception Centre, and general practitioners. Voluntary agencies which have borne our questioning include, amongst many others, Alcoholics Anonymous, Al–Anon, Giles House, St. Luke's House. Rathcoole House (Alcoholism Recovery Project), which is reported on in an article by Mr Timothy Cook, has been financed by the Carnegie Trust, the Home Office and King Edward's Hospital Fund. It owed its inception to the imagination and energy of the late Dowager Marchioness of Reading, and its success to the residents, staff, house committee, and the local officers of Social Security, who together built and supported this experiment.

Certain authors and co-authors who have not at any time been staff members of the Research Unit have generously allowed their work to be published in a book emanating from the Unit. In this regard we would thank Dr E. Brown, Dr Peter Cole, Mr Timothy Cook, Dr D. L. Davies, Dr Bert Falkowski, Dr C. Feyerabend, Dr Denis Gath, Professor Michael Gelder, Dr Brian Hore, Dr Michael Kelly, Dr Gelhin Morgan, Mr E. Myers, Dr Benno Pollak, Professor Michael Shepherd and Dr Terence Spratley.

Research of the sort we report in this book relies fundamentally on the generosity and trust of people who owe the research workers nothing, and who answer what must often seem intrusive questions. In this regard our thanks must by now be due to many thousands of individuals – we will not attempt here to categorise them, but to each and every such person we express our gratitude for their helpfulness and tolerance.

Expert statistical advice and help with data processing has been given at different times by Mr Michael Brown, Miss Jane Chandler, Mr Michael Clark, Miss Margaret Elliott, Mrs Hedi Firth, Mr Christopher Hayes, Miss Carole Hewlett, Miss Barbara Kinsley, Professor A. E. Maxwell, Mr Peter Nicholls, Mrs Frances Parsons, Mr Upendra Patel, Mr Julian Peto, Dr Patrick Slater, Mr Colin Taylor, and staff of the Department of Biometrics of the Institute of Psychiatry, International Computers and Tabulators Ltd., the London School of Economics, and the University College Computer Centre.

The secretarial staff of the Unit have always been full members of the research team, and we wish to acknowledge their skills, energy, patience and unstinting loyalty. The following gave help in the original preparation of published papers: Miss K. Blick, Miss Nadine Butler, Mrs H. Cooper, Miss E. Cross, Mrs S. Ghosh, Miss Christine Guest, Miss Pauline Hampson, Mrs S. Heaven, Mrs Laura Hitchins, Mrs Joy Hodge, Miss Marion Horton, Mrs Gaynor Impanni, Mrs Joyce Oliphant, Mrs Julia Polglaze, Miss Sue Rees, Mrs Jean Crutch, Miss Pat Bevan, Miss Serena Dalrymple, Miss Jacqueline May and Miss Beryl Skinner. Mrs Sylvia Ghosh has played a central part in preparing the present book for publication.

The Unit's survey work has over the course of years been assisted by the services of many temporary interviewers. In other aspects of our studies we have received generous practical help from medical social work and record staff of the Bethlem Royal Hospital, the Maudsley and various other hospitals.

Messrs May and Baker kindly supplied the Metronidazole and placebo used in one investigation reported here.

We would thank the Editors of the following journals for permission to reprint material which appears in this book: *British Journal of Addiction, British Journal of Preventive and Social Medicine, British Journal of Psychiatry, British Medical Journal, Lancet,* Nacro Papers and Reprint Series, *Psychological Medicine, Quarterly Journal of Studies on Alcohol,* and *Social Psychiatry.*

We thank the journals concerned and the authors for waiving copyright fees. All royalties from the sale of this book will be paid to the funds of the Addiction Research Unit.

To our publishers thanks are due for unfailing helpfulness and much patience.

Preface

This book puts together a number of research reports on drinking and smoking which have over recent years come from the Addiction Research Unit of the Institute of Psychiatry. The final section presents five essays which bear on what has been called here the research position, and which deals with particular aspects of the working life of a research unit, and the responsibilities of the research worker. Also in several instances authors who have not been members of the Unit's staff have generously contributed to this volume.

For any one research centre to suppose that its own work is worthy of being assembled in book form is temerity. Other things go on in addiction research besides the work of the ARU, and this both in Britain and internationally. By the time work is published in a journal its referencing is probably not up to date, and a collection of already published papers is inevitably lacking in the excitement of the just published report.

Despite these reservations which must apply to any exercise in the general art form of 'collected papers', there seemed on due consideration to be a place for putting together in this book the Unit's work. The whole is more than the part, and the hope is that this volume may present not only an assemblage but also a perspective. The picture which it is hoped to convey is of the type of questions which inter-disciplinary research can ask, the sort of methods which it can employ, the problems and frustrations it will encounter, and all this in much larger measure than any pretence that this volume presents resounding new truths.

The sections and sub-sections of this book are each given a short introduction simply by way of sign-post. Each part of the book is then rounded off by an appraisal, which seeks to identify the underlying and unsolved questions which the papers throw up.

This volume will have served its purpose if it excites criticism, and most importantly if it arouses the critical interest of social and behavioural scientists. The sad fact is that up to the present in this country the main-stream of sociology and psychology has paid scant attention to alcoholism and smoking. There have from various centres been distinguished individual contributions but this only serves to underline the general lack of any continued tradition of academic regard for this area. If anyone claims a concern that social science should be socially relevant, the study of why people by the hundreds of thousands damage themselves with these socially accepted drugs, and the study also of why the social acceptance, are beckoning areas for research.

A companion volume presents some of the Unit's work on proscribed drugs (opiates, cannabis and amphetamines), and examines some theoretical perspectives. At the scientific level there is need for research and thinking which throws down 'substance barriers' and which encourages emergence of theories of substance-seeking behaviour applicable across the whole spectrum of alcohol, nicotine and other drugs. And at the levels of public attitude and policy there is need for an awareness that there can be no absolute and comfortable distinction between alcohol bought at the pub, the packet of cigarettes from the corner shop, the bottle of tranquillisers prescribed all too casually by the doctor and the miscellaneous substances of illicit use. It is the illicit drugs which capture the attention of the media but it is alcohol and tobacco which on any rational basis must be seen to constitute by far the larger part of 'the drug problem'. The two volumes of the Unit's work which are now published deal not with different problems but with facets of the same problem.

DRINKING STUDIES

1 Introduction

The section on drinking studies is divided into three parts. The first group of papers describes a survey of the drinking habits of a sample of the general population of a London suburb, and a survey of student drinking. The focus here is on drinking more than on abnormal drinking, although such surveys will in passing give some measure of drinking problems.

The second clutch of papers is concerned with another epidemiological approach, and this is the study of special groups and estimates of alcohol-related morbidity in high prevalence groups. The characteristics of the Unit's researches have in this aspect no doubt been determined by its location: the Unit has alcohol-related casualty on its doorstep. Camberwell has within its boundaries the largest reception centre for homeless men in the country, and two large prisons lie just outside those boundaries. Camberwell Green is a short walk down the road, and in all but the coldest weather there will be a scattering of Skid Row men sitting on the park benches.

In the third part of this section the papers deal with treatment and determinants of treatment outcome, the work reflecting the close relationship between the Unit (and its parent Institute), and the Bethlem Royal and Maudsley hospitals. Assessment of treatment methods and design of treatment approaches has been seen from the Unit's beginning as one research priority, but a research concern with hospital treatments has been tempered by awareness that with alcoholism the hospitals can only be part of the helping response, with the contribution by voluntary community organisations continuing in this country to play a most important role. The final part of the alcoholism section therefore presents research on community organisations, and on that most important community agent, the alcoholic's spouse.

Part I Surveys of drinking behaviour

2 Drinking in a London suburb*

GRIFFITH EDWARDS, ANN HAWKER, CELIA HENSMAN,
JULIAN PETO and VALERIE WILLIAMSON

Summary

This paper reports on a survey of 'normal drinking'. Interviews were conducted on a sample of 928 adults living in a South London suburb. Typical class patterns of drinking were identified, and the difference between the drinking of men and women (with class interaction) stood out clearly. Both for men and for women three motivational factors were identified, with a basic similarity between the factors for the two sexes. For both sexes an 'ataractic' motivational factor (drinking to relieve unpleasant affect) was associated with heavier drinking and higher trouble score. The disparity between male and female prevalence of trouble with drinking was marked, especially for high trouble score categories.

2.1 Introduction

(a) *The problem of describing drinking behaviour*

There is no single measurement which adequately describes a man's drinking. If only the quantity of his intake over a given time is recorded, very different forms of behaviour will appear to be identical: a man who drinks 14 pints of beer in a week may have drunk two pints every day of that week, or he may have consumed all 14 pints on the Saturday night. Similarly, a description of frequency alone cannot give an adequate representation. The obvious solution to this dilemma is that originally proposed by Straus and Bacon (1953): by

---

* A condensed presentation of material originally published in the *Quarterly Journal of Studies on Alcohol,* Supplement No. 6, 1972, pp. 69–93, 94–119, 120–8.

reference both to the usual quantity of alcohol consumed by the individual on a drinking occasion and the usual frequency of his drinking, the subject is placed in one of a number of QF (Quantity–Frequency) categories.

QF categorisation was in the present survey based on enquiry into each subject's drinking of 15 types of alcoholic beverage during the 12 months prior to interview. For each beverage questions were directed at:

(a) *Frequency,* with the eight forced-choice categories: every day, most days, weekends only, once or twice a week (not limited to weekends), once or twice a month, once or twice in six months, on special celebrations only or once or twice a year, never.

For any beverage which the subject admitted to having drunk during the previous 12 months, further questioning was directed at:

(b) *Usual quantity* in terms of 'usual upper limit during the last 12 months on one drinking occasion'. Quantities were coded in units, with half-a-pint of beer, a single of spirits and a glass of wine taken as equivalent to one unit.

The beverage selected as the one on which the individual's QF categorisation was made, was the beverage for which the subject gave the highest frequency rating. If two beverages rated equally for frequency, the beverage rating highest on usual quantity determined categorisation. Using the selected beverage, each subject was then assigned to one of the six possible QF categories:

1 *Abstainer.* Admitted to no alcohol at all consumed during the previous 12 months.
2 *Occasional.* F was not more than once or twice in six months. Q might be any amount, but inspection of data showed in fact that low frequency were almost without exception also low quantity subjects.
3 *Infrequent light.* F was once or twice a month and Q was taken as up to three pints of beer (or equivalent) on a usual occasion.
4 *Frequent light.* Once or twice a week or more frequently, with up to three pints of beer on a usual occasion.
5 *Moderate.* This category embraced those who drank moderately and frequently, and those who drank heavily but only moderately often.
6 *Heavy.* A subject placed in this category drank more than three pints of beer at a usual sitting, and drank at least once or twice a week.

The major limitation of the QF approach was found to be that the highest category embraced a very wide spectrum of behaviours indeed, and the analysis was therefore in some instances supplemented by analysis of *total week's alcohol intake* (in equivalent of pints of beer), reconstructed for the seven days prior to interview.

6

(b) *Sampling and interviewing*

Sampling was within each of six housing estates in one London borough and was chosen to give a wide socio-economic spread. There were no houses in multiple occupancy: problems of subject location which might confront the interviewer were thus much eased, but at the same time the decision not to include multiple occupancy or slum property inevitably excluded a potentially interesting group. In each estate approximately one in three households were chosen by sampling within units of similar rateable (city tax) value. All subjects aged over 18 years who were usually domiciled in these chosen households, were then to be interviewed. On 89 per cent (928) of subjects successful interviews were completed. Thirty-eight per cent of all interviews were conducted by four permanent staff members of the research team, while the remaining 62 per cent were carried out by 15 interviewers specially hired and trained for the purpose.

(c) *Demographic description of the sample*

Results in this sub-section are given as *percentages* of the 928 subjects interviewed, unless otherwise stated. The data aim simply to establish certain important general features of the population studied.

Male 44, female 56.
Age 18–25 11; 26–35 18; 36–45 22; 46–55 17; 56–65 18; 66–75 9; 75+ 5.
Single 17, married 68, widowed 12, divorced or separated 3.
Church of England 69, Roman Catholic 18, Nonconformist 5, Jewish 3, none 3, other 2.
English 86, Irish 5, Scottish 2, Welsh 1, other white 5, non-white 1.
Full-time employment 54, part-time 16, housewife only 22, retired 6, ill or
    unemployed 2.
Social class by Registrar–General's classification by occupation (General Register Office 1966): I (professional) 4; II (technical) 15; III (skilled) 44; IV (semi-skilled) 18; V (unskilled) 18.
Place of birth: London 70, other UK 23, overseas 7.

2.2   Description of normal drinking

Demographic features and QF categories

1   *Male and female QF distribution.* Males tended to be heavier drinkers than females (P. <.001), as exemplified by only 24 per cent of males as opposed to 46 per cent of females being abstainers or occasional drinkers, while 14 per cent of males and less than one per cent of females were in the

heavy drinking category.

2　*Sex and social class.* In Table 2.1 the distribution between QF categories shows significant class difference both for males (P. <.001) and, combining moderate and heavy categories, for females (P. <.001).

Closer inspection suggests the importance of a sex/class interaction in determining drinking behaviour and the following comments can be made:
(a)　Social Class I, II. The most striking characteristic of the drinking of these classes is that approximately half of both men and women are placed in the frequent/light category. There are differences between male and female drinking but the differences are in general less marked than in III, IV or V. Both among men and women abstention is rare, while 27 per cent of II men go into the moderate or heavy category compared with 46 per cent of III males, 46 per cent of IV, and 40 per cent of V. The general statement can therefore be made that in QF terms I, II females tend to be heavier drinkers and I, II males lighter drinkers than subjects in other classes.
(b)　Social Class III, IV, V. In each instance the commonest category for men is moderate, and male drinking does not differ dramatically as between these three classes. There are no very striking between-class differences here as regards the females either, but for all three classes there is the strong and consistent trend for heavier male than female drinking.

3　*Sex and age.* Younger age groups drink more heavily than older and distribution between QF categories is significant both for men (P. <.001), and combining moderate and heavy categories for women (P. <.001). The cumulative influence of sex and age is sharply illustrated by contrasting the 55 per cent of young men (aged 18–34) who are moderate or heavy drinkers with the two per cent of 50+ women who are placed in those categories.

4　*Sex and religion.* Comparing simply the largest two denominational groups (Church of England and Catholic) among males there is a significant tendency for RC subjects to be heavier drinkers (P. <.05), but among women (combining moderate and heavy categories) the tendency, although in the same direction, is not significant.

5　*Sex and nationality.* Nationality was defined in relation to a father's nationality. Scottish and Irish combined, both men (P. <.05) and women (P. <.01), are more heavily represented among the heavier drinking categories than are the English and Welsh.

Parental drinking and QF categories

Subjects were asked to categorise each parent's drinking as abstainer or special occasion only/ordinary social drinker/quite heavy or too much.

1　*Father's drinking.* For male subjects (combining QF categories 2, 3, 4)

Table 2.1

QF categories according to sex and social class

QF CATEGORY	Social Class															
	I and II				III				IV				V			
	male		female		male		female		male		female		male		female	
	n = 81		n = 97		n = 176		n = 228		n = 78		n = 85		n = 67		n = 98	
	n	%	n	%	n	%	n	%	n	%	n	%	n	%	n	%
Abstainers	3	4	2	2	12	7	20	9	3	4	12	14	9	13	16	16
Occasional	12	15	23	24	35	20	105	46	12	15	30	35	10	15	25	26
Infrequent/light	6	7	18	19	14	8	43	19	13	17	15	18	5	8	22	22
Frequent/light	38	47	48	49	34	19	42	18	14	18	22	26	16	24	29	30
Moderate	15	18	6	6	51	29	16	7	24	31	6	7	18	27	6	6
Heavy	7	9	–	–	30	17	2	1	12	15	–	–	9	13	–	–

there is a significant difference (P. <.01) in QF category distribution as between the different parental categories. The percentage of subjects of heavy QF increase in step with heavier parental category – 8, 15, 24 per cent. For female subjects (again combining same QF categories), the corresponding difference in distribution is again significant (P. <.001). The relation here is however certainly not a simple one: the daughters of fathers who are 'ordinary social' drinkers tend to drink more heavily than those whose fathers are placed in either of the extreme categories.

2 *Mother's drinking*. For male subjects mother's drinking exerts no significant influence while for female subjects QF category distribution (using category combinations) is significantly influenced by maternal drinking (P. <.05). The number of women in QF 2–5 (i.e., drinkers as opposed to abstinent or near abstinent subjects) increases stepwise – 51, 60, 75 per cent – with heavier maternal category.

Scores on Eysenck personality inventory and QF categories

Each subject completed the short form of the Eysenck personality inventory (Eysenck and Eysenck, 1964) which rates both E (extroversion) and N (neuroticism) on a scale of 0–6. Both for males and for females higher QF categories tend to have higher mean E scores (e.g., male abstainers mean E = 2.8, QF 6 mean E = 4.7). Neither for males nor females is there a consistent relationship between QF and mean N score.

Usual beverage, sex and QF categories

As in determining the F of the subjects' QF category, 'usual' beverage was the one given the highest frequency rating by the subject, with the beverage choice defined here as 'multiple' in the case of a tie. Heavier drinkers tended toward a beverage choice typical of their sex, which for men was beer and for women spirits.

Sex, class and influence of the weekend

The weekend exerted strong influence on the drinking behaviour of subjects of both sexes and of three social class groups with the exception only of males of Class I–II (Table 2.2). This latter segment shows itself less influenced by the weekend than any other group, though even here wine drinking shows some patterning. Class I and II women do not share this emancipation to the same degree as their menfolk.

10

Table 2.2

Sex, class and influence of the weekend: percentages of subjects drinking on stated day.

Subjects in Class I, II n = 82, III n = 177, IV, V n = 146 for males; Class I, II n = 97, III n = 230, IV, V n = 182 for females.

	Males			Females		
	I–II	III	IV–V	I–II	III	IV–V
Sunday	50	48	40	40	26	29
Monday	57	25	21	32	8	8
Tuesday	50	27	15	33	9	8
Wednesday	51	23	16	27	8	8
Thursday	55	27	14	25	7	7
Friday	56	36	21	25	11	11
Saturday	60	47	40	46	24	27

Sex, class, and frequency of drinking in different settings

(a)   *Males.* Significant class differences exist for each setting. The pub is the preferred place of drinking – 'usually' or 'always' for 37 per cent of Class I, II but for 60 per cent of III and 61 per cent of IV, V; drinking in the home is preferred by 34 per cent I, II, but only by 13 per cent of III and 9 per cent of IV, V, while never drinking in the home shows the converse class relationship; drinking in other peoples' homes is class related in much the same way as drinking in own home; drinking in restaurants is a very strongly class related habit – 73 per cent of I, II would do so at least sometimes, while for III the corresponding figure is 28 per cent and for IV, V 9 per cent.

(b)   *Females.* Significant class differences again exist for each setting and resemble those seen with men. It is in use of the pub that men and women most sharply differ in choice of drinking setting: about half as many women as men (whatever the class) will give the pub as the preferred setting, and regardless of class about one quarter of women who drink will never use the pub.

Discussion

1   *Implications for the understanding of normal drinking*

The results of this survey show that it is impossible to describe a 'typical' drinking pattern of 'this suburb' – there are typical drinking *patterns* related

11

both to class and sex. There are many possible explanations, some speculative and some which appeal to commonsense.

(a) *Patterning by money.* Drinking focused on the weekend is, for instance, very probably dictated by the weekly pay-day.

(b) *History.* Fully to understand a pattern which can be observed today may well necessitate understanding the pattern from which it was derived. It would seem possible that the eighteenth and nineteenth century drinking among the poor of this country has left its legacy of patterns and traditions, albeit there has been much change.

(c) *Drinking as definition of status.* Certain modes of drinking which may once have been determined by identifiable social or economic causes are later perhaps invested with secondary and perpetuating symbolic importance.

Demographic factors are however not the only variables which are correlated with drinking behaviour. The finding that extraversion but not neuroticism is associated with higher QF is reminiscent of the similar finding with cigarette smoking (Eysenck, 1965). In that there may be a hereditary contribution to extraversion (Shields, 1962) and that father and son will also often tend to resemble each other in social class, the findings regarding the relationship between parental and subject's drinking behaviour are not easy to interpret. That father's but not mother's drinking is related to the drinking of the male subject does however suggest the possible importance of identification with the parent in determining drinking habits.

2 *Implications for the understanding of abnormal drinking patterns*
It would seem likely that 'extrapolation' of I, II drinking would lead typically to quite a different type of problem than would extrapolation of III, IV, V drinking. Class I and II 'frequent light' drinking would have as its natural progression frequent and heavier drinkers; an unremarkable slippery slope would lead to the type of alcohol intake which induces dependence or cirrhosis. In contrast, the likeliest progression of III, IV, V 'heavy' sporadic drinking, might be towards heavier sporadic drinking and hence drunkenness and disturbed behaviour.

3 *Implications for prevention of abnormal drinking*
The contrast between the drinking pattern of the I, II male and the IV, V female make it starkly obvious that any taxation, education, or other social manipulation which has as its imagined target the 'typical British drinker' can do no more than discharge a blunderbuss. Before the preventive expert gets to work he clearly therefore has to ask himself what type of drinking, in what particular sub-culture, he is trying to transmute into some other drinking pattern – and this transmutation with what potential harm as well as with what benefit?

12

2.3   Comparison of male and female drinking motivation

This section is concerned with stated motivation for drinking by 306 men and 281 women from the total sample who drank 'once or twice a month' or more often. The 17 questions on motivation were:

1   I drink because I like the taste.
2   I drink because I get thirsty.
3   I drink because it makes me feel good.
4   I drink because it helps me to relax.
5   I drink when things get me down.
6   I drink because it helps me to sleep.
7   I drink because my job demands it.
8   I drink because it helps me to forget my worries.
9   I drink because it's difficult to refuse.
10   I drink to celebrate, or on holiday.
11   I take a drink for health reasons.
12   I drink because it goes well with meals.
13   I drink sometimes when I'm restless or tense.
14   I drink to liven things up when they are dull and boring.
15   I drink because other people are drinking.
16   I drink because it revives me and makes me feel ready to face things.
17   I drink because it's a habit.

To each question each subject gave a yes/no response.

Results

1   *Percentage of subjects answering affirmatively to each motivation question*
There were only four items (numbers 2, 7, 14 and 17 of the above list) on which female and male answering rates differ significantly (all at P <.001) and in each instance it was a matter of women giving lower rates than men.

   Both for women and for men the rank ordering shows an intermingling in the sequence of social and personal reasons, such that it would be difficult to make any general and common-sense statement as to one or other type of motivation being consistently the more popular.

2   *Factor analysis of female motivation and of male motivation separately*
The method used for the factor analyses is described by Lawley and Maxwell (1963). The factor analysis of male motivation has been described in detail elsewhere (Edwards et al., 1972a). Table 2.3 gives factor loadings both for

13

women and for men. The first female motivation factor will be referred to as F1, the first male as M1, and so on.

(a) *First factors.* F1 and M1 show remarkably similar loadings. They indicate a type of motivation related to drinking which is for the relief of unpleasant effect and may conveniently be termed '*ataractic*' factors.

(b) *Second factors.* In the previous analysis of male motivation, M2 was seen as reflecting drinking which is done for '*sophisticated*' reasons, and with women there is again high loading on drinking for taste and drinking with meals. In other respects F2 and M2 appear to be roughly parallel but there are also some important differences. This sort of comparison by eye can be misleading, though, and it is probably best simply to regard F2 and M2 as picking up different but (in commonsense terms) overlapping motivation.

(c) *Third factors.* F3 and M3 again show some similarities but also some dissimilarities. F3 and M3 both to some extent reflect motivation which is a response to social pressure, or '*clubbable*' motivation.

3 *Correlation of factor scores with other variables*

Correlations between factor scores, personality factors, age and week's total alcohol consumption were explored. The following comparisons can be made between the sexes:

(a) Total week's alcohol consumption is for the males very significantly correlated with the first factor, and for that sex, week's drinking is correlated significantly with no other factor. For women the week's consumption shows a correlation with the first factor which is still very significant but lower than for the men; for the women the second factor is in this regard slightly (but not significantly) more important than the first. The week's consumption shows a slight but significant negative correlation with N for women and with E (positive) for men.

(b) F1 just fails to show a significant correlation with N while M1 shows a very significant correlation.

(c) Age shows very significant negative correlation both with F1 and M1, and also with F2.

4 *Factor scores and social class*

(a) *First factors* both for women and for men show no significant or consistent class relationship.

(b) *Second factors.* F2 shows a class relationship which is consistently uni-directional (high I, low V), while M2 shows significantly higher mean in classes I and II than in the other groups.

(c) *Third factors.* F3 shows no class relationship, while M3 is consistently uni-directional with higher means in the lower status groups.

5 *Factor scores and trouble scores*

A 'trouble score' was calculated for each individual as the sum of his or her

14

Table 2.3
Factor analysis of female motivation and of male motivation separately.
Factor loadings <0.300 by an asterisk

Variate	First factors		Second factors		Third factors	
	Female (F1)	Male (M1)	Female (F2)	Male (M2)	Female (F3)	Male (M3)
1 Celebration or holiday	-0.013	-0.046	0.382*	0.091	0.106	0.171
2 Taste	0.099	0.007	0.390*	0.437*	-0.130	0.071
3 Relax	0.535*	0.506*	0.220	0.329*	-0.083	-0.057
4 Other people	0.000	-0.102	0.074	-0.086	0.356*	0.436*
5 Feel good	0.375*	0.407*	0.274	0.240	-0.009	0.298
6 Meals	0.130	0.012	0.395*	0.463*	-0.033	0.054
7 Thirsty	0.167	0.038	0.255	0.306*	-0.147	0.356*
8 Difficult to refuse	-0.053	0.205	-0.113	0.010	0.419*	0.538*
9 Health problems	0.126	0.188	-0.280	0.013	-0.125	-0.084
10 Things get me down	0.729*	0.687*	0.015	0.100	-0.129	0.048
11 Restless or tense	0.585*	0.562*	0.212	0.113	0.038	0.028
12 Dull and boring	0.424*	0.411*	0.091	0.075	0.152	0.401*
13 Revives me	0.621*	0.423*	0.023	-0.032	-0.081	0.136
14 Sleep	0.499*	0.461*	-0.281	-0.160	0.067	0.074
15 Forget worries	0.585*	0.677*	-0.103	-0.081	0.030	0.094
16 Habit	0.221	0.156	0.000	0.075	0.405*	0.264
17 Job demands	-0.075	0.032	0.152	0.427*	0.143	0.013
% variance accounted for	15.52	15.53	5.06	5.47	3.56	4.20

affirmative answers to a list of 25 questions which were concerned with untoward drink-related happenings (see section 2.3 of present paper) occurring during the 12 months prior to the interview.

(a) The first factors for both sexes show consistently higher means with progressively higher trouble score categories; differences are significant.

(b) For women the second factor also shows this tendency but the differences between means are small and not significant. For men there is no consistent trend.

(c) The third factor for women shows a consistent trend with larger differences between means, but the variance is such as to make confident interpretation difficult. For men there is no consistent trend.

Discussion

The relationship between true motivation and the answers obtained by this sort of verbal report procedure remains problematical. Only a small part of the variance has so far been accounted for. With these reservations in mind, two provisional conclusions would seem to be in order:

1 The motivational structure which actuates female and male drinking seems to be roughly similar.

2 For women and for men these three different motivational factors may however be of rather different significance, a state of affairs which may well alter as the culture permits increased drinking by women. With men it is the first factor (ataractic) which stands out as most strongly related to quantity drunk and to trouble experienced; with women the first factor is still of generally similar importance but the female second factor is a more important correlate of quantity drunk and the third factor possibly important as a predictor of trouble. With women it is interestingly the third rather than the first factor which gives a significant (but small) correlation with N score.

Cross-national and cross-sex studies of drinking motivation might prove illuminating in terms of what they revealed as to the ability of different cultures to model or control the behaviour of the person who might, from stated motivation, be expected to be at risk of developing trouble with drinking.

2.4 Differences between male and female report of drinking problems

The present section compares reported occurrence of specific 'trouble' items by men and women: the nature of these items is shown in Table 2.4 and it can be seen that the word 'trouble' is being used to indicate a range of occurrences from the trivial to the severe.

16

Table 2.4

Troubles with drinking during the last 12 months in men and women, in percentages. The percentages in columns 1 and 2 are rounded to the nearest whole number (< 1 denoting less than 0.5 per cent), while the ratios are calculated from the unrounded numbers.

	Men (N=408)	Women (N=520)	M:F Ratio	P
After drinking have you found your hands shaky in the morning?	7	3	2.5	.01
After drinking have you ever found you can't remember the night before?	6	3	2.5	.01
Have you ever been 'under the influence'?	25	9	2.7	.001
Has your doctor ever advised you not to drink as much as you do?	2	1	3.2	.05
Have people annoyed you by criticising your drinking?	5	1	3.5	.01
Have you ever gone without drink for a period to prove you can do so?	8	2	3.7	.001
Have you ever had health problems due to drinking?	2	< 1	5.1	.05
Have you ever felt you ought to cut down on your drinking?	8	2	5.4	.001
Have you ever had fights with family or friends after drinking?	3	1	5.9	.01
Have you ever had trouble or quarrels with family or friends because of your drinking?	5	1	6.1	.001
Have you ever had a drink first thing in the morning to steady your nerves or get rid of a hangover?	4	1	6.4	.001
Have you ever arrived late at work due to a hangover?	6	1	8.0	.001
Have you ever missed a day's work because of a hangover?	3	< 1	8.9	.001
Do you ever find that when you start drinking you can't stop?	2	< 1	11.5	.01
Have you ever spent more money than you ought to on drink?	8	1	13.2	.001

All percentages take the successfully-interviewed 408 men and 520 women as base, except where otherwise stated.

1 *Occurrence of particular troubles during the previous 12 months*
In Table 2.4 items have been rank-ordered so that those with lower male/female ratios appear toward the upper part of the table; for ten additional items the women gave zero report. There is no item for which the male reporting rate is not more than twice the corresponding female rate, and for nine items which give low (< 1 per cent) report by males, the females report no occurrence at all. It is also obvious that the male/female ratio varies greatly from item to item (2:5 to 13:2), but in many instances with only very small numbers being involved in calculation of ratios, it would be a mistake to read too much into the precise ratio for any individual item.

2 *Occurrence of four or more times of certain troubles during the previous 12 months*
When frequency of occurrence over fixed time was enquired into, rather than simple presence or absence of occurrence, such an approach by and large increased the apparent male/female disparity.

3 *Summed trouble scores*
Trouble scores for each individual were calculated by totalling all those items which that subject had experienced once or more during the previous 12 months. The disparity between male and female report increases with severity of trouble category, and for the problem drinking category (operationally defined as occurrence of five or more trouble items during the 12 months) the male/female ratio was 8:0. Indeed, among the 520 women interviewed, only four were identified as problem drinkings, (males 25) with the extreme female trouble score reported being seven (male extreme score 18).

4 *Categorisation of subject by previous week's drinking*
Taking the parameter of previous week's total alcohol intake as illustrative, a drinking behaviour variable and trouble scores can then be cross-tabulated (Table 2.5). It is apparent that men and women who drink the same quantity experience no significant difference in trouble, while the virtual absence of any women from the heaviest drinking category is mirrored by the very low report of serious trouble by women. The bottom line of the table seems to go some way toward explaining the difference between male and female experience of drinking pathology but the question is really, of course, only shifted back to a more basic question – we have it seems to ask not why women experience less trouble but why women drink less.

5 *Correlates of trouble with drinking*
With men there is a tendency for higher trouble scores to be significantly

Table 2.5
Alcoholic beverage consumption by men and women, in percent and mean
trouble score in consumption groups

Consumption in pints/beer or equivalent in last 7 days	Men (N=408)	Women (N=520)	Mean trouble score	
			Men	Women
0	29	51	0.4±0.3	0.1±0.1
0.5–5	33	40	0.5±0.2	0.3±0.1
5.5–10	17	9	0.9±0.4	0.7±0.4
10.5–15	8	1	1.3±0.7	1.5±2.0
Over 15	13	0.2 (N=1)	3.7±1.1	1.0

associated with higher N (neuroticism) scores, but to be unrelated to E (extroversion).

The small numbers of women in the higher trouble score categories are generally accompanied by a wide scatter on any scores which describe the characteristics of those women; the relationship between TS and N is similar to that seen in the males but there is also some relationship between TS and E. Relationship between TS and motivational factors has been discussed in Section 2.3 of this paper.

The strongest hypothesis to explain differences in male and female problem rates seems on present evidence to be that this difference is to be understood as very closely related to the underlying sex difference in normal drinking patterns. Such a hypothesis is then consistent with another finding – the male/female ratio for drinking pathology is found to depend on the chosen definition of pathology, and tends to be greater when the definition implies more serious pathology. Such accords with the finding that male and female percentage representation in any drinking behaviour category diverges more widely, the heavier the drinking. The fundamental question then seems to be whether females drink less (and hence experience less trouble) because of constraints on drinking itself, or because of prohibition imposed on problematic behaviour; the two matters are likely to be closely related, but are not identical. It would also be of interest to know how far such constraints are a matter of external control and how far they are introjected and sensed as personal value.

Drinking pathology must then, besides, be seen in the wider context of male/female differences in deviant or pathological behaviours in general. The literatures on crime, mental illness, suicide, drugs and smoking throw up so many parallels with the problems which surround understanding of male/female differences in drinking behaviour, that one may indeed wonder whether the traditional demarcation of research areas is altogether helpful. Understanding of differential alcoholism rates may in the end be dependent on understanding of general and basic matters related to societal definition of sexual differentiation.

Between-sex studies are less costly and less difficult to set up than transcultural studies, but may indeed provide very similarly useful research opportunities. A reason for supposing that research focused on the sex differential may deserve quite high priority is that, in many parts of the world, the social definition of the man's and of the woman's place is becoming subject to large changes. Must female emancipation carry with it an inevitable steep rise in female alcohol dependence?

3   Drinking in a London suburb: reinterview of a sub-sample and assessment of consistency in answering*

GRIFFITH EDWARDS, CELIA HENSMAN and JULIAN PETO

Summary

Eighty subjects from the original 'normal drinking' sample were reinterviewed after an interval of two to three months. Drinking behaviour measures gave fairly high consistency but factor analytical motivation variables gave poor reinterview consistency. Relationship between variables ('structure') was fairly consistent.

Method

(a)   *The Sample.* The original interviews were conducted on 408 men and 508 women, and the sampling method for that occasion has been described (Edwards et al., 1972a). For reinterview a sample of 40 men and their wives (80 subjects) was selected.

All reinterview subjects were not only married but also currently living with spouse, and aged 40–65 years. On first interview all had been co-operative on first or second contact. The sub-sample was broadly representative of the original group in terms of housing status.

(b)   *Time lapse.* Subjects were reinterviewed within two to three months of the original occasion.

(c)   *Questionnaire.* The questionnaire was a shortened version of the original: its content is apparent from the headings in the 'Results' section of this paper.

(d)   *Interviewers.* Four interviewers who had been employed on the original survey each now interviewed 20 subjects who were not among those whom the particular research worker had interviewed on the first occasion.

---

* Synopsis of a paper of the same title originally published in *Quarterly Journal of Studies on Alcohol,* vol. 34, 1973, pp. 1244–54.

Results

1 *Variables other than those relating to subjects' drinking*

(a) *Religion in which brought up.* Eight subjects (ten per cent) stated a religious affiliation different from that at the first interview.

(b) *Father's nationality.* In only one instance (one per cent) was this item unreliable.

(c) *Father's drinking.* A five-point categorisation was used on each occasion (Edwards et al., 1972a). In 61 cases (76 per cent) answers were identical on the two occasions. In only one instance (shift from I to IV) was there major inconsistency.

(d) *Mother's drinking.* In 63 cases (79 per cent) there was consistency, and in no instance a shift involving more than one category.

(e) *E (extraversion) and N (neuroticism)* as measured on the short form of the E.P.I. (Eysenck and Eysenck, 1964). Correlation (roe) between first and second interview was 0.80 for E and 0.71 for N.

2 *Subjects' drinking behaviour*

(a) *Number of days out of seven days previous to interview on which any drink at all was taken.* The correlation was 0.76 and difference of more than one day occurred in 16 cases (20 per cent).

(b) *Usual drinking quantity (Q).* The question related to 'usual upper quantity on one drinking occasion during the last 12 months', and results were converted to units equivalent to half-pints beer. Using three-pint brackets, in 62 cases (77 per cent) there was consistency, while in only four instances was there a change of more than one bracket.

(c) *Usual frequency (F) of drinking during last 12 months.*
This was categorised in terms of:
I   Every day or most days.
II   Weekends only or once/twice per week.
III   Once/twice per month or less.

There was complete consistency in 66 cases (82 per cent), and in no instance was the shift more than one category.

(d) *Quantity-frequency (QF) categorisation.* Subjects were placed in one of the five QF categories (Edwards et al., 1972a).

In 54 cases (67 per cent) there was complete consistency while in seven cases (nine per cent) there was inconsistency of more than one category. There was no consistent tendency for higher QF placement on one occasion, but among the higher categories (QF III, IV), the tendency was for lower placement on second than first occasion (nine subjects, 11 per cent) rather than vice versa (three subjects, four per cent).

3 *Adverse effects of drinking*

A 'trouble score' (Edwards et al., 1972b, c) was on each occasion calculated by simple summation. The correlation was 0.66, but the complete consistency of 51 cases (64 per cent) was largely accounted for by the 44 subjects (55 per cent) who gave zero trouble scores on both occasions. Six subjects (8 per cent) were inconsistent by two or more points, and this was all in the direction of lesser admission on the second than the first occasion.

4 *Motivation for drinking*

(a) *Procedure.* Factor analysis using the method described by Lawley and Maxwell (1963) was performed on the data obtained on the first interview occasion from all those 587 subjects who gave a drinking frequency of once a month or more. The factor loadings were closely similar to those obtained on previous separate male (Edwards et al., 1972d) and female (Edwards et al., 1974) factor analyses, with factor loadings in all instances falling between the corresponding male and female loadings. These factors were, as before, identified as: *factor 1,* 'ataraxic motivation'; *factor 2,* 'sophisticated motivation'; *factor 3,* 'clubbable motivation'.

Factor scores for the 52 subjects in the reinterview sample who had on either first or second occasion stated a drinking frequency of once a month or more, were then calculated for first and for second occasion.

(b) *Consistency of factor scores.* For the 52 reinterviewed subjects, correlations on first and second occasion were for first factor 0.56, for second 0.66, and for third 0.61.

(c) *Consistency of relationship between factor scores and other variables.* The majority of correlations were similar on first and second occasion, e.g., correlation of first factor with week's total consumption 0.512 on first and 0.545 on second interview data. The relationships were also generally very similar to those seen in the original reports with separate-sex analysis correlations.

Discussion

1 *The study's design*

Extrapolation from this sub-study to the likely level of consistency which would have been revealed if the whole original sample had been reinterviewed is not permissible, and present results are best considered as simply indicating an 'order of magnitude'.

Some of the questions (e.g. demographic) asked, were such that shift could only be susceptible to explanation in terms of error. Whether changes in N and E scores are inevitably to be interpreted wholly in terms of error, must depend on whether these variables are to be seen as somewhat fluctuating attributes.

Turning to items where shift might be explained both in terms of error and of true alteration, the basic drinking behaviour variables all show that roughly 70 per cent of subjects may be expected to give the same answer twice. The Q and F questions applied to drinking during the 'previous' 12 months: the period of overlap would be nine to ten months. It is difficult to believe that the shift is other than largely error. Trouble score questioning similarly applied to 12 months, and it again seems unlikely that the major contribution to the shift can be other than error.

That both as regards the higher QF categories and as regards trouble scores the shift was towards lesser admission on the second than the first occasion should be noted.

The relatively low correlations between first and second measures of motivational variables constitute prima facie evidence for supposing that these measures are to a degree unreliable, and that there is particular need for research investment which will build reliable instruments for assessment of motivation.

Table 3.1

Trouble score categories and mean motivation
scores for first and second interview occasion

Trouble score category	First Interview		Second Interview	
	N	First factor mean	N	First factor mean
0	30	−0.27	33	−0.47
1–2	15	−0.23	14	−0.38
3–	7	+0.38	5	+0.38

3   *Consistency of relationships between variables*

The degree of consistency of relationship between variables as seen on the first and then on the second occasion, and in particular the consistency of relationship between first factor score and week's drinking and trouble scores, is in accord with the notion that survey work of this sort can reliably reveal basic structural relationships.

4   Drinking behaviour and attitudes and their correlates amongst English university students*

JIM ORFORD

Summary

A self-completion questionnaire was returned by 1,323 students (75 per cent response). Principal component analysis was carried out on 18 variables and two major components identified. Independent 'problem drinking' and 'social drinking' variables were not identified. Individual anxiety level may modify drinking to a degree, but a much more important determinant is peer-group influence. Women drank in a relatively more 'restrained' manner than men.

The structure of the drinking domain

Each student was assigned a score on each of 18 variables on the basis of replies to questions concerning drinking behaviour and attitudes. These items covered the following areas: recent drinking frequency and quantity; style of drinking in terms of type of beverage, place and company; tolerance; perceived motivation; psychological effects of drinking; attitudes to self and others drinking, and self and other drunkenness; reported concerns and complications regarding drinking; reported experience of intoxication and 'morning after' effects.

These variables were intercorrelated for three samples separately (males at one college; males at the second college; females) and the three correlation matrices subjected to factor and principal component analyses. The principal component analyses showed the greater consistency between samples. The intercorrelations were almost uniformly significant and positive and for all three samples there was a large first component to which nearly all variables contributed, which accounted for approximately 40 per cent of the total variance. The second ranking component, in order of size, accounted for very much less of the variance (eight to ten per cent) and appeared to contrast a greater experience of and interest in drinking, as against a greater experience

---

* A paper specially written for this volume giving a summary of a study fully reported in the *Quarterly Journal of Studies on Alcohol* in 1974 (vol. 35, no. 4, pp.1316-74).

of and interest in the psychological effects of drinking and drunkenness. 'Problem drinking' variables had higher loadings on the first component than on the second. Further components accounted for less of the variance, were less consistent between samples, and more difficult to interpret.

Two conclusions about the structure of the drinking domain for these student samples would appear to be warranted:

1   The relative sizes of these components suggest that individual differences in terms of *general overall interest in drinking* (component 1) are much more prominent amongst students than are individual differences in terms of *relative interest in drinking per se vs. drinking for psychological effect* (component 2).

Answers to the questions: 'how much do you drink?' or 'how much do you like drinking?' tell very much more about the nature of a student's involvement in drinking than would answers to the question: 'in what way do you drink?'

2   The results confirm a previous failure to discover independent 'problem drinking' and 'social drinking' dimensions for students (an unpublished Ph.D. thesis by Park, 1958).

There is no support in these findings for the view that differences between 'healthy' and 'unhealthy' patterns of youthful drinking are very prominent and important, and it might be suggested that programmes of alcohol health education for the young based on this assumption are unlikely to be very successful.

Personality and social influence correlates of drinking components

Each student was also assigned a score on each of six personality variables (extraversion, neuroticism, a lie scale score, adventurous pleasure-seeking, radicalism, tender-mindedness) and on each of five social influence variables (report of father's drinking, mother's drinking, friends' drinking, perception of father's approval of the student's drinking; perception of mother's approval). Scores on each of these variables were correlated with scores on each of the two principal drinking components.

General overall interest in drinking (component 1) had highest correlations with the personality variables of extraversion and adventurous pleasure-seeking, particularly with the latter variable. High scorers on the scale of adventurous pleasure-seeking, designed specially for this study, were more likely to report that they dated frequently, smoked a lot, drove fast and had broken the law and were less likely than other students to report going to church. Neuroticism, or anxiety, had much lower correlations with the first component but higher for females than for males. General overall interest in drinking was correlated significantly with all five social influence variables but when the effects of the other variables were partialled out, friends' drinking (as reported by the student himself) was the only one still significantly correlated. The magnitude of these partial correlations between scores on the first component and friends' drinking were the highest obtained in the whole study (0.45 to 0.56).

There were few significant correlations with interest in drinking *per se* vs. drinking for psychological effects (component 2). However, neuroticism, or anxiety, was significantly associated with an interest in drinking for psychological effect, although the correlations were small in size (0.16 to 0.28), while adventurous pleasure-seeking was significantly associated with interest in drinking *per se,* but for male students only.

It would appear that, although anxiety level may modify students' motivations for drinking somewhat, there is much more support for the conclusion that student drinking is very largely under the control of peer group influence, and if personality or temperament are influential they are influential in the form of individual differences in sociability and interest in involvement in a variety of adventurous pleasure-seeking activities.

Sex differences

Comparisons between male and female students were made for each of the individual drinking behaviour and attitude variables employed in the study, as well as for many of the individual items. Males were found to score significantly more highly on nearly all individual variables and items whether they referred to drinking quantity and frequency, interest in drinking, attitudes towards drinking or reported intoxication, complications due to drinking or concern about drinking. Within this general picture of sex differences, however, some variables produced more dramatic sex differences than others and some surprisingly produced virtually no sex differences.

Male students differed from female principally in being much more likely to admit to drinking large quantities of alcohol (five pints of beer or the equivalent, or more) occasionally (although in terms of 'average' quantities sex differences were much smaller); in sometimes drinking medium or large quantities quickly; in being much more likely to drink in the company of members of their own sex only; in being more likely to take the initiative on drinking occasions; in reporting complications attributable to drinking which involved conflict with people in authority (being involved with the police and being reprimanded by such people as teachers or employers). On the other hand, female students were just as likely to admit to having felt guilty about their drinking, to having made a decision to stop drinking altogether even if they later reversed the decision, and to having been frequently reprimanded about their drinking by a friend. Furthermore, although the differences are not statistically significant, female students advocated a slightly higher ideal frequency of drinking for their age-sex group than did male students for theirs; were slightly more likely to admit drinking for effect; were slightly more likely to admit that they experienced psychological effects from their drinking; and reported slightly more frequent drinking of wine, drinking with parents, and drinking with meals.

It is very tentatively suggested that women may be just as much motivated towards, and may just as often experience, the mood-modifying properties of alcohol as a drug, but the different rates of alcoholism or problem drinking for the sexes which have been so frequently reported may be attributable to the relatively 'restrained' and 'constrained' manner in which women tend to drink, which is itself attributable to the prevailing norms of sex-appropriate behaviour.

5   Appraisal

Why undertake drinking studies of this type? Such work is expensive and time-consuming at the stage of field-study, and the multivariate problems presented at the analysis stage constitute a notorious headache. The answers to be given to this question are at least three in number.

First, there is simply the scientific opportunity presented and the scientific challenge. The immediate content of the research is drinking behaviour, but drinking behaviour is really only taken as a convenient examplar of the generality of socially/psychologically determined behaviour. If the science of social-psychology has anything to offer, then surely this is exactly the sort of field in which it ought to demonstrate the strengths of its techniques and research strategies. And as for the multivariate problems, far from these being an unwelcome complication of this sort of research, they might be seen as a welcome and practical opportunity for exploring what statistics has to offer the social sciences; in this regard it may be noted that the techniques employed in the final reporting of the data generated by these two studies, represent only the end product of a great deal of analytical trial and error by statisticians who were enthused by the problems and generous of their time.

If there was a particular lesson underlined by this research it was that co-operation with the statisticians has to be at every stage, and that research planning which puts the analysis stage under unfair time-pressures is self-defeating. The demands of funding sometimes seem to mean that the full richness of what might be got out of the data is sacrificed to guilty anxieties generated by the feeling that it is high time that particular project was all tied up and the team re-deployed on the next project. There should be time to live with data, juggle with it, and play with it in any number of ways. To this extent the conventional teaching that the analytical plan should be built into the research design is insufficient; there are always unexpected and alternative ways of giving meaning to the data.

The second reason for undertaking surveys of this sort might be seen as the low-level and practical one of obtaining minimum prevalence estimates of pathology; however defined, this may correct society's perceptions and serve to make the basic debate as to the appropriate level of society's concern rather better informed. The results of the adult drinking survey are used to this end in another paper which appears in the present book.

Thirdly, it might be argued that research of this type might actually contribute to the design of a rational basis for preventive strategies. This is a much more daring expectation, and the results so far obtained obviously provide only very tentative leads: what these leads might be is to an extent discussed in the papers themselves.

So much for an attempt to answer the initial awkward questions – a statement of purposes. There are then many unanswered questions which relate to methodology. The reliability and validity of data obtained from this type of enquiry is widely open to question although reinterview of a subsample of the adults involved in the first study gives not altogether discouraging results. The literature however gives no room for complacency and drinking in any survey is undoubtedly going to be under-reported, with different biases probable at different drinking levels. Measures of drinking motivation require much refinement, and any team which would sufficiently invest in this problem to build a standard and reliable instrument would be giving a valuable gift to the research world. Orford's analysis of 'the drinking domain' also highlights the fact that, as regards drinking behaviour, there are a great variety of possible questions, but still much uncertainty as to which of these questions are those worth asking: his suggestion that questions really group themselves into just two important areas is obviously worth further study.

Any research team which has dabbled in drinking surveys must indeed come away from the experience with a chastened awareness of the difficulties. One is asking people on a large scale about matters that they may be loath to admit, unable to remember, or in the case of motivation unable satisfactorily to articulate. The concept of 'motivation' is here itself in many ways unsatisfactory. To say all this is not to preach nihilism. There can be no doubt as to the importance of the questions which the survey method attacks, and even with the present relatively crude approaches some of the truths and relationships may be strong enough to come through. One must conclude however that survey research at present sets up a large agenda for methodological studies which must refine the tools of the trade, and drinking surveys in this regard do not of course stand alone.

Part II Surveys of special groups

6   London's Skid Row*

GRIFFITH EDWARDS, ANN HAWKER, VALERIE WILLIAMSON
and CELIA HENSMAN

Summary

A sample of 51 men drawn from the regular patrons of a soup kitchen in Stepney were interviewed. Mean age was 44.7; 64 per cent were Irish or Scottish; 74 per cent were Roman Catholic; the background was predominantly that of low socio-economic status and 58 per cent had in childhood experienced some degree of parental deprivation. The typical adult life-style was one of social instability and social isolation. As for drinking, 49 of the 51 men were alcohol dependent. The logistics of Skid Row are described, and the group's previous treatment and criminal history. Implications for treatment are discussed.

Introduction

In most parts of London today it is rare to see a man drunk in the street. Certain localities are, however, still frequented by broken-down inebriates. The areas by the Elephant and Castle and Waterloo in South London remain among the chief haunts of these men, while in the East End, the Stepney and Aldgate districts have their Skid Row. Filthy and dishevelled, with face often blackened by the smoke of the fires which are lit in derelict houses or on bombed sites, the Skid Row alcoholic is not difficult to recognise.

Several studies have been published in this country on the type of alcoholic who is admitted to the specialised psychiatric units. In the series reported by Davies et al. (1956) and Glatt (1961a) the proportion of middle-class patients was high; and a similar social background was found among members of Alcoholics Anonymous (Cooper and Maule, 1962; Edwards et al., 1965). In

---

* This paper was originally published in the *Lancet*, vol. 1, 1966, pp. 249–52.

contrast, little is yet known of the characteristics of the population that make up London's Skid Row. This is surprising, for in America the same problem has been extensively studied (Pittman and Gordon, 1958) and it was this aspect of alcoholism which in the 1940s first persuaded sociologists that abnormal drinking was a proper subject for scientific investigation (Straus, 1946; Straus and McCarthy, 1951). The American sociologists evolved the 'under-socialisation hypothesis' – the hypothesis that the origins of alcoholism are to be found in the patient's inability to put down social roots or to become responsive to social control – but it was soon realised that this was a too sweeping generalisation, and that the derelict inebriate made up only a small part of the total alcoholic population (National Council on Alcoholism, 1959).

We have carried out an enquiry to diagnose the nature of the disorder which leads men to the bombed sites and to surgical spirit drinking, and to see whether the diagnosis can suggest action more rational and more constructive than the present policy of repetitive short-term imprisonment.

Method

The sample consisted of 51 men drawn from the regular patrons of a soup kitchen in Stepney. The vagrants who come there are mostly alcoholics and the majority are known personally to the clergyman and to his helpers who provide the free, hot evening meal. We asked the clergyman to go into the canteen and to ask the first man whom he encountered (and whom he knew to be a heavy drinker) to agree to an interview. There was a ready willingness to co-operate due, partly, to the trustful and friendly relationship between the canteen staff and the vagrants and partly to the men's gratification in finding that research workers should be interested in their lives. Anyone interviewed was given a packet of cigarettes.

All of the cases but four were found indeed, to be men with drinking problems. Two were rejected from the sample as not really heavy drinkers, one was found not to be a drinker at all but to be a compulsive gambler, and one was not an alcoholic but a barbiturate addict.

The questions usually required specific answers but some allowed for more scope in reply.

Three interviewers (AH, VW and CH) were social workers with experience of alcoholism research and interviewing techniques and the fourth (GE) was a psychiatrist.

The background

Characteristics of the sample

The mean age was 44.7 years (range 26–74). The biggest group were of Irish origin (37 per cent), while Scottish (27 per cent) and English (26 per cent) were almost equally represented. The preponderance of Roman Catholics (74 per cent) was striking and is not accounted for simply by the Irish contribution. No-one had been brought up in free churches and there was no Jew.

Family background and childhood

The fathers were predominantly of low socio-economic status; but sufficiently detailed information could not be obtained to make an accurate classification in terms of the Registrar General's social classes.

There were 29 (58 per cent) cases in which the subject was during childhood, for a period of three or more years before the age of 13, deprived of a continuing relationship with one or with both parents. The majority of the sample came from large families (average sibship 5.4). Eight had been before juvenile courts for a variety of offences ranging from stealing apples to arson.

The average age on leaving school was 14.2 years. Only eight had gone to school beyond the age of 14 and none had had higher education.

Adult social stability

Contact with relatives. Only three men had communication with any relative during the previous year. Twenty-five stated that they had had no contact for five or more years. Among these were 14 men who had severed contact for more than ten years.

Marriage. Seventeen had been married once and one had been married twice. In every instance the marriage had broken irrevocably. In three instances the wife was said to have had a parent who was a problem drinker, and three men stated that their wives were alcoholics.

Occupation and working stability. Few men had ever acquired occupational skill – one had trained as an electrician, one had been a tarpaulin maker, one had been a tailor, two had been clerks, and one man stated that he had been 'a stockbroker in the Dominions'. Fourteen had been merchant seamen, the remainder had never done anything but unskilled labouring. Only two – the tarpaulin maker and one of the clerks – had ever held a steady job for five years or more.

Period of greatest social stability. Thirty-four subjects (67 per cent) had never achieved any stability at all since leaving home — if they had married, they had never really settled down to live with their wives, and they had never been able to find a job and hold it. The other 17 (33 per cent), however, had for generally rather brief periods, attained some roots — often this was in the interlude between discharge from military service and setting off on a drifting career.

The road to Skid Row

Average ages have been calculated (Table 6.1) as a rough guide to the sequence of events which takes a man ultimately to the bombed sites, but they are not strict 'steps' followed in every instance by every case. Some men have never been to prison at all, and many have never been in a mental hospital.

Symptomatology of pathological drinking

The symptoms of 29 men who drank 'crude' (surgical or methylated) spirits and of 21 men who either never touched crude spirits or turned to this source of supply only very occasionally, are analysed in Table 6.2. One surgical spirit drinker did not answer these questions.

The morning symptoms of nausea, shakes, sweats, craving and blackouts for the previous night and day-time amnesias were recorded with no significantly greater frequency among the crude spirit drinkers than among the others, but the last three symptoms were experienced with greater severity in the crude spirit drinking group; for these three symptoms the distribution between 'slight' and 'severe' categories is significantly different ($P < 0.05$) when the two groups of drinkers are compared.

Table 6.1
Milestones on the way to Skid Row

Milestones	Average age (yr.)
Drinking regularly	18.2
Drinking most days	23.6
Drinking heavily	25.2
Drink a problem	29.0
First drunk arrest	29.3
First imprisonment	33.5
On Skid Row	38.0
First hospital admission	41.5

Table 6.2

Symptomatology of pathological drinking; comparison between crude spirit and other drinkers

Symptom	Regular drinkers of crude spirit (29)			Other drinkers (21)		
	severe	mild	total	severe	mild	total
Morning nausea	7	20	27	9	10	19
Morning shakes	8	20	28	9	8	17
Morning sweats	11	14	25	10	6	16
Morning craving	4	23	27	8	9	17
Morning amnesia	5	20	25	9	6	15
Day amnesia	5	16	21	6	3	9

The two groups differ in hallucinatory experience but not at the five per cent level (Table 6.3). Auditory hallucinations were more frequent in the crude spirit drinkers: 14 had experienced the symptom in conjunction with visual hallucination, and seven had experienced auditory hallucination alone, so that in total 21 of the 29 surgical spirit drinkers (72 per cent) reported auditory hallucinations, whereas only nine out of 21 (43 per cent) of the other group had experienced this symptom. In frequency of visual hallucinations, the two groups did not differ.

How many of these men would be considered 'gamma alcoholics', in Jellinek's classification (1960)? When the schedules were examined in detail

Table 6.3

Hallucinatory experience: comparison between crude spirit and other drinkers

Hallucinatory experience	Drinkers of:	
	Crude spirit (29)	Other alcohol (21)
Both auditory and visual	14	6
Only auditory	7	3
Only visual	2	5
Auditory alone or in combination	21	9
Visual alone or in combination	16	11

the answer was usually clear – a group of symptoms was present which would put the diagnosis of 'gamma alcoholism' beyond doubt in 49 out of 51 cases (96 per cent).

In the Skid Row culture hallucinatory experience was considered 'normal', and the hallucinatory nature of this experience was recognised with insight. The auditory hallucinations were sometimes interpreted as being due to 'ghosts', but beyond this there was no secondary elaboration. In contrast, the visual hallucinations were often terrifying. These too, however, were an accepted occurrence. One man, when asked if he had ever 'seen things' answered 'naturally'.

Drinking habits

Men were more likely to drink in a gang than alone, but gang drinking was significantly more frequent in the crude spirit group.

Crude spirit drinking

In every instance except one, the man had been introduced to this form of alcohol by another person offering him crude spirit; and the occasion was often vividly remembered. The usual story was of a man being penniless and unable to find the price of the pint of cider or bottle of wine which he was desperately needing to alleviate his withdrawal symptoms, and of his then being charitably given a swig from someone's bottle of surgical spirit. The number of different cities in which the first experience had taken place gives some hint as to the widespread nature of the Skid Row problem – London, Manchester, Nottingham, Ely, Southampton, Swindon, Glasgow, Belfast, and towns in Canada were mentioned.

Seven subjects stated that they preferred crude spirit to any other form of alcohol, but the others all said that they drank crude spirit only because it was cheaper. Each man was asked whether crude spirits produced any effect which ordinary drink could not give. All but one said this was so, but the men had difficulty in saying precisely what it was about crude spirit which made the experience special.

Of the 30 crude spirit drinkers, two never drank methylated spirits but always took surgical spirits, and one drank methylated spirits exclusively. Eight out of the 30 crude spirit drinkers always took the drink neat; the remainder used a variety of diluents such as water, lemonade, or, very occasionally, wine. Four men mentioned that it was their habit to start the day with the spirit undiluted ('raw') and when this had 'taken the sickness off them' they would dilute the remainder.

The average quantity of crude spirit drunk a day was 2.2 pints (44 oz.) either as methylated spirits (2s.2d./11p a pint) or surgical spirit which was generally bought for 2s. a pint.

Refusal by chemists to sell surgical spirit had been encountered by 23 men, but there were several shops well known for their laxity. Gang drinkers wanting surgical spirits would often overcome the shopkeeper's unwillingness by sending the least dishevelled member of the gang to make the purchase – one man stated that he had never bought his own drink. Buying methylated spirits was in contrast always easy: hardware stores were reported to be 'not in the habit of asking questions'. Methylated spirits was also obtained from garages (sometimes at inflated prices).

Fifteen men had at times experimented with other forms of de-natured alcohol, or with other intoxicants.

Choice of drink among those not drinking crude spirits

It was not usually possible to gauge the individual's total daily average alcohol consumption – the choice and combination were so variable that no simple estimate could be made. Often a man would drink whisky – or rum or gin – if he were rich, and if not so well-off drink a cheap wine. Wine or a cheap sherry cost about 8s. per bottle, and men would drink two or more bottles of this per day. If money were not available for wine, then rough cider was the next choice, and anything up to 20 pints a day would be consumed. Beer was a more expensive alternative to cider, and more of it had to be taken to produce the same effect. One man stated that he could drink up to 40 pints of beer a day, but he was much in the lead: three men claimed 25 pints of beer a day.

The logistics of Skid Row

Money

Each man was asked how he had obtained money during the previous seven days (Table 6.4). In general a man had obtained money from more than one source, and the totals in the table therefore add up to more than 51.

'Welfare sources' in Table 6.4 means National Assistance, unemployment money, and sickness money. The reason why more men did not claim was their difficulty in stating a fixed address and on occasions men would go into a hostel for no other reason than to establish an address. Of the seven pensions, six were ex-service and one was an old age pension.

Thus out of 51 subjects, 47 (92 per cent) had found enough money for their week's needs without any regular employment.

Table 6.4
Sources of money during previous week

Source of money	No. of men
Casual work	15
Borrowing	8
Begging	16
Welfare sources	14
Pensions	7
Pooling with gang	21
Pawning or selling	4
Discharged prisoners' aid	2
Pilfering	5
Other charities	5
More regular employment (kitchen work)	4

Accommodation

Of the 51, 32 (63 per cent) had not during the whole of the previous week had one night's shelter other than that provided by derelict dwellings.

'Sleeping rough' may mean the bombed houses, but these men also at times slept in telephone booths, all-night laundrettes, air-raid shelters, parked cars, and all-night cafés.

Thirty (59 per cent) of the men were 'barred' from various hostels in London.

Food

Men were questioned on what they had eaten during the 24 hours before the interview. Only two had eaten anything approaching a substantial meal.

Movements

Of the 51 men, 28 spent nearly all their time in the East End and 18 frequented the Elephant and Castle or the Waterloo area and loyalty to a particular area could become quite partisan. In the summer many of these alcoholics would move off to find kitchen work in the hotels of coastal towns.

Other history

Drug taking

Experimentation with drugs had been common but true dependence rare. Two men had taken cocaine for a brief period and one stated that, many years previously, in Canada, he had been a heroin addict. Drug experimentation had been more frequent among the crude spirit drinkers than among the remainder: 11 crude spirit drinkers had at one time tried 'purple hearts' and only three of the others had experimented with this drug, while ten of the spirit drinkers had some experience with benzedrine and only one of the others. Five men had tried reefers and one had tried barbiturates. Benzedrine seems to have enjoyed favour in the days when inhalers were easily bought, but the general view was that drugs, compared to alcohol, had little to offer. Several men when asked about drug taking expressed fiercely moralistic views.

Physical illness

Eight men had had a peptic ulcer diagnosed at a hospital and four of these had undergone gastrectomy. Four men had been treated for pulmonary tuberculosis. Besides one man who, as a child, had lost a leg in an accident, three had lost both legs as a result of accidents in adult life. Four had had severe leg fractures and one had sustained a fractured pelvis.

Suicidal attempt

Ten had attempted suicide and seven of these were surgical spirit drinkers. It was clear that many of these attempts had been manipulative or demonstrative gestures.

Admission to mental hospitals

Twenty men (39 per cent) had at some time been admitted to either a mental hospital or an observation ward and between them these 20 totalled 46 separate admissions: the greatest number of admissions for any one man was seven. Of the 46 admissions, five were to observation wards. Fourteen men stated that they had at various times attempted to get treatment for their drinking and been refused admission.

Arrest and imprisonment

Forty-seven of the 51 admitted to having been arrested for drunkenness.

Forty men had been in prison. Twenty-one had been in gaol less than ten times, and 19 had been in more than ten times. The information here was so confused and complex that it was difficult to know with certainty whether criminal activity had started before drink became a problem, although prison records were checked in all cases for which these were available: the general impression gained was that only a minority had been in any trouble before their drinking. Thirteen had at some time attempted, unsuccessfully, to get arrested, hoping thereby to get a week or two's shelter in prison.

Length of time on Skid Row

Only 40 subjects could be included in the analysis since it was not always easy to decide with certainty when a man could be considered to have arrived on Skid Row. Of these 20 had been on Skid Row for less than three years. (The scatter was wide with an 'average' of 5.7 years).

The demand for help

Each man was asked 'If you were offered the chance to go into hospital for treatment of your drinking problem, would you accept this help'? Thirty-two men said they would accept (17 crude spirit drinkers and 15 others). Some men, although wanting help, felt that hospital was not the place.

Validity

The difficulty of assessing the validity of information gained by interviewing vagrant alcoholics, many of whom have much to conceal, is clearly considerable. Our general impression was, however, that these men seldom prevaricated and were astonishingly open in their answers. We stressed that if there were questions they did not want to answer, they should simply say so rather than give an untruthful answer.

Discussion

Diagnosis

The explanation of alcohol addiction put forward today is that, although alcohol is a weak drug of addiction, enough taken for long enough will induce a biochemical change in the body which is then the physical basis for a syndrome of pharmacological dependence. This syndrome is preceded by years of heavy drinking originating in psychological factors and social pressures rather than in any metabolic disease. Does this hypothesis explain Skid Row, or is the vagrant drunk not to be considered a 'real' alcohol addict?

42

Without doubt all these men were addicted to alcohol and chemical dependence had been established in severe form. The appalling severity of withdrawal symptoms shaped a pattern of life devoted to ensuring supplies of alcohol, with all other motivation forgotten.

What then were the factors responsible for the heavy drinking in this group which preceded the addiction? The adult inability of these men to find roots seems to have been caused in the first instance not by their drinking, but by their damaged personalities, and the origin of this damage could often be seen in a childhood home where the benefits of human contact were scant indeed. To define the personality disorder narrowly, as if there were a 'Skid Row personality', would be spurious, but among the elements of the disorder were often restlessness, irritability, and profound difficulty in forming rewarding emotional contact. This disorder not only set a man drifting but invited him to quiet his malaise by drinking.

How is this multifactorial explanation of the aetiology to account for the very special way in which these addicts have ended up, i.e., their arrival on Skid Row? Part of the answer is perhaps that they are there because little existed to stop them from getting there — they came from loosely knit working-class families which would evince little concern for a deviant member and would readily let him drift out of contact. In contrast, the tendency of the middle class to rescue its distressed members must often obstruct progress to Skid Row.

A man's arrival on Skid Row is not, however, due only to his path thither being unobstructed; an important part of the explanation is that he took that path because the whole Skid Row milieu answered so many of his needs. He has found a pseudo-adjustment which makes his anxieties tolerable; he has opted out of the society which demands close emotional engagement and which expects him to make decisions and bear responsibilities. The nature of Skid Row has not been fully understood until it has been seen not simply as the chaotic end-result of addictive drinking, but as a way of life which fulfils the needs of a damaged personality. The vagrant alcoholic has worked out a pathological adjustment but an adjustment none the less: he is institutionalised on Skid Row.

The diagnosis of Skid Row is thus threefold: a life-long personality disorder, an acquired chemical disease, and a pathological social adjustment.

Treatment

The diagnosis dictates the treatment. The primary illness from which the Skid Row alcohol addict is suffering is a personality disorder which cripples his ability to adjust to a normally demanding life. If the aim is 'cure' then the therapist is going to be frustrated: a stay in a mental hospital or a course of treatment in a specialised alcoholism unit can have only trifling impact on this grossly damaged personality, and can do little to improve the man's ability to face the world on the day on which he leaves hospital. The whole approach, however, becomes rational and optimistic when the aim is seen not as cure of an illness but as the support and rehabilitation of a patient with irrevocable defect.

Support, as we have already suggested, may be what Skid Row itself provides. The basis of rehabilitation must be to offer lifetime hostel care with the hostel designed specifically to satisfy the emotional needs of this group of men, and to be even more aptly suited to their needs than was Skid Row. Something must be created with a magnetism which pulls more strongly than the old draw of Skid Row. Such an atmosphere does not come about by chance, but requires for its creation skilled staff who are able to control and exploit group processes. Dependency on the hostel and on its staff must be accepted and even encouraged. Treatment here means to have on offer a less pathological adjustment than institutionalisation on Skid Row, and therapeutic skills lie in designing an adjustment which these types of personality can use. The therapist must stay close to reality.

Part of the diagnosis is also, however, a severe drug addiction and although the long term hope is that dependency on the hostel can to some extent replace dependency on alcohol, frequent relapse into drinking will for many men be inevitable. A clearly stated policy on what happens to a man when he drinks is essential, and the least anxiety provoking policy, both for the group and for the individual, seems to be that if a man drinks he immediately leaves the hostel, but that later readmission is never refused. Group discussions similar to those conducted by Alcoholics Anonymous can be helpful, and 'Antabuse' (given under proper medical supervision) should probably be given routinely.

A blue-print for such a hostel has been produced by the Camberwell Council on Alcoholism, [1] but there is already ample evidence for the practicability of such an approach from Myerson's pioneering experiment in America (Myerson, 1956). Even if judged only in cash terms, a hostel, with residents who are working and contributing to their keep is less of a burden on the taxpayers than having the vagrant alcohol addict chronically unemployed, destitute, begging, dependent on welfare, absorbing the energies of police and magistrates, and repeatedly imprisoned.

The results of this investigation suggest that many of the men on Skid Row would accept a place in a supportive hostel without compulsion. The exact percentage who would reject aid cannot of course be assessed until help is there to be refused; for this residium some change in the law or some re-interpretation of the Mental Health Act may ultimately be necessary to enforce long term care in a closed institution. Wider use of compulsion, however, cannot be justified either in terms of humanity or economics until enough hostels have been built to provide those who want help with the help they need.

Note

[1] The ideas put forward in that blue-print were translated into reality when in 1963 the Alcoholism Recovery Project opened Rathcoole House, Clapham.

7 Census of a reception centre*

GRIFFITH EDWARDS, VALERIE WILLIAMSON, ANN HAWKER, CELIA HENSMAN and SETA POSTOYAN

Summary

Two hundred and seventy-nine residents of a large statutory shelter for homeless men (reception centre) were interviewed. Demographic background, etc., is described. Not less than 25 per cent were on crude criteria showing evidence of alcohol dependence, while 45 per cent had at some time been arrested for drunkenness. In other respects the heterogeneity of the population was striking and the great variety of life problems with which they were faced. Implications for the future planning of community care are discussed.

Survey procedure

Britain's statutory reception centres (of which 19 existed in 1965) give free accommodation to the destitute and are increasingly involved in rehabilitation. Camberwell has the biggest such centre in the country.

A 100-item structured questionnaire was after preliminary piloting administered by a team of 22 interviewers to 279 men who were resident in the Camberwell Reception Centre on the night of 28 April 1965.

Results

1 Demographic

Age: Mean age was 46.1 (SD 12.2) years.
Marital status: Seventy per cent of men were single, 1 per cent married with marriage considered intact, 16 per cent separated, 8 per cent divorced and 4 per cent widowed.
Ethnic origin: Country of birth was England 51 per cent, Ireland 20 per cent, Scotland 14 per cent, Wales 5 per cent, other white culture 6 per cent, non-white culture 4 per cent, (including 1 per cent West Indian).

---

* Synopsis of a paper of this title originally appearing in the *British Journal of Psychiatry,* vol. 114, 1968, pp. 1031–9.

Social class: Distribution of social class of subjects ('best ever') was 3.5 per cent Class I, II; 22 per cent III, and 72.5 per cent IV, V, (remainder unknown), by the General Register Office (1960) classification.

2   Social stability

Within the previous six months men had on average spent at the longest 14.1 weeks (standard deviation 8.7) in one place of residence. Eighty-two per cent were unemployed.

3   Physical illness

Thirteen per cent stated that they had suffered from a peptic ulcer, eight per cent had been treated for tuberculosis, 11 per cent had been in a general hospital during the previous six months.

4   Mental illness

The number of times men had been in a mental hospital (for reasons other than drinking) was 0, 76 per cent; 1, 13.5 per cent; 2, 5.0 per cent; 3, 2.5 per cent; 4, 1.5 per cent; 5 or more 1.5 per cent. Seven per cent had been in a mental hospital during the previous six months.

5   Drinking

Hospital treatment: eight per cent had at some time received inpatient and two per cent out-patient hospital treatment for drinking.
Drink a problem: nine per cent of subjects saw drink as 'at present' being a problem, and 30 per cent saw it as a problem either now or in the past.
Symptoms of pathological drinking: see Table 7.1.

Table 7.1
Occurrence rate (percentage) of symptoms of abnormal drinking

Symptoms	Percentage			
	Never	'Once or twice'	'Quite often'	'Unsure'
Morning amnesias	62	12	24	2
Morning shakes	61	10	25	4
'Morning livener'	60	9	28	3
Arrest for drunkenness	53	'Ever' 45		2

Table 7.2

Correlation between different indications of drinking pathology

	'Drink a problem now'	IP	Morning drink	Amnesias	Morning shakes	Drunk arrest	Usual beer	Usual wine	Usual spirit
In patient ever for drink	.524								
Morning drinks ever	.530	.344							
Amnesias due to drink ever	.546		.528						
Morning shakes ever			.651	.554					
Arrested for drunkenness	.423		.446	.438	.449				
Usual quantity of beer				.318		.321			
Usual quantity of wine	.433		.452	.369	.367	.304			
Usual quantity of spirit			.331	.318	.350			.498	
Surgical spirit ever	.338							.337	

Drunkenness arrests: those who had been arrested for drink (45 per cent of total) had on average been arrested 8.5 times, but there was a wide scatter (SD 14.5): 22 per cent of those arrested had only been so once, but 21 per cent had undergone arrest more than 20 times.

Correlation between different indicators of drinking pathology: these correlations are set out in Table 7.2, only those greater than .3 are shown, and these are all significant beyond the .001 level.

6 Imprisonment

Fifty-nine per cent of men had at some time been in prison, and 18 per cent had been in prison during the previous six months.

Discussion

What in essence is the picture of the reception centre population which emerges from this research? The really striking feature is the heterogeneity: rather than the data adding up to make one whole picture, it seems that pieces of several different puzzles have been thrown together. Under one roof are being performed the functions of an old people's home, lodging house for the itinerant labourer, alcoholism rehabilitation centre, mental after-care hostel, half-way house for the discharged prisoner, and perhaps a dozen other functions besides. Small specialised hostels might offer a much better hope of effective rehabilitation than the present large and confusedly multi-purpose reception centres. Hostel care is at the forefront of thinking in many different fields, and inevitably, the Government may some time have to consider the possibility of a hostel service (*British Medical Journal*, 1966).

8　Drinking problems in a prison population*

GRIFFITH EDWARDS, FRANK GATTONI, CELIA HENSMAN and
JULIAN PETO

Summary

A five-point 'dependence score' is described, with its rationale derived from
learning theory. Alcohol dependence is thus conceived as existing in degrees,
rather than its being all-or-none. Taking a recidivist prison population as the
sample for study, degree of alcohol dependence is related to criminal
behaviour, aspects of drinking behaviour, and indicators of general social
instability. The prevalence of drinking problems in the prison population is
determined in relation to a variety of definitional criteria; different definitions
lead to widely different answers. Drinking problems certainly show greater
prevalence among short term than long term prisoners. Implications for
policy are briefly considered.

Introduction

In 1965 the research team set up a survey in a recidivist prison. The sample
consisted of 188 short term (sentence three months or less), and 312 long term
prisoners (serving sentences of one year or more), with sampling for each
group simply on basis of consecutive admission. Interviews were conducted
by prison officers who received special training. Special emphasis was put on
the independent research nature of the exercise and subjects knew that their
answers could have no bearing on their sentences. The interview schedule was
based on an 80-item questionnaire previously employed in a study of a
reception centre (Edwards et al., 1968).

The results of the survey will be presented in two parts. In the first section,
the concept of a 'dependence score' is developed, and the idea applied in some
detail to the short term group. The second section then looks at this and other

---

* This paper adapts material contained in the two following previously
published reports: 'Drinking problems among recidivist prisoners',
Psychological Medicine, vol. 1, 1971, pp. 388–99, and 'Correlates of alcohol
dependence scores in a prison population', *Quarterly Journal of Studies on
Alcohol,* vol. 33, 1972, pp. 417–29.

measures of drinking pathology prevalence, as applied both to short and long term groups.

8.1 Correlates of dependence scores in a short term recidivist population

The relevance of physiological dependence to an understanding of the nature of alcoholism is uncertain. The alcoholic drinks excessively long before he develops the shakes, and the physiological phenomena can therefore be interpreted as no more than rather unimportant happenings along the way, as epiphenomena rather than as essence of dependence. A different interpretation and one which derives from Wikler's hypothesis on the implications of operant conditioning for understanding of dependence (Wikler 1961, 1968) gives, on the other hand, considerable weight to the importance of withdrawal symptoms in the genesis of alcohol dependence. Whatever the potency of the straightforward euphorogenic effects of alcohol as a reinforcer of alcohol-seeking behaviour, its reinforcing property will (it could be argued) become vastly more potent when it has not only a primary psychotropic property, but now also the secondary property of relieving withdrawal distress. This model may embrace also the idea of dependence being in part a conditioned avoidance of low blood alcohol levels which prelude withdrawal; withdrawal symptoms are not envisaged as being-and-essence of dependence, but as providing a mechanism which allows the building of much stronger operant conditioning than can usually come from primary euphoria alone. Dependence is not then seen as an all-or-none phenomenon: the severity of dependence is to be judged by the strength of a conditioning process.

The two opposing evaluations of the withdrawal syndrome can in summary be placed in this contrast. The first sees the physiological syndrome as *caused by dependence,* while the latter sees the physiological syndrome as *importantly contributing to the establishment of dependence.*

This latter view of the significance of the withdrawal syndrome does seem to propose hypotheses which are testable, e.g.:

1   The intensity of dependence might be measured by a scale which took account of frequency with which the withdrawal syndrome had been experienced and frequency with which it had been relieved by drinking.

2   With other factors (e.g., class) more or less equal, the degree of social disability might be related to degree of dependence.

Such hypotheses could of course be tested on any alcoholic population and there is as ever the problem of no available population being truly 'typical'. The analysis which follows relates to data obtained from the 188 short term recidivist prisoners – a population which is highly unrepresentative of the generality of drinkers in this country, but which has the advantage of

51

containing a wide spectrum of drinking behaviours and a high prevalence of supposedly drink-related problems.

Dependence scale

Each subject was rated on a five-point scale in terms of affirmative answers to the following questions:

1 'Have you ever woken up with your hands very shaky as a result of a previous night's drinking?'
(a) 'Never'   Score 0
(b) 'Just once or twice'   Score 1
(c) 'Quite often'   Score 2
2 'Have you ever taken a morning drink to steady yourself after a hard night's drinking?'
(a) 'Never'   Score 0
(b) 'Just once or twice'   Score 1
(c) 'Quite often'   Score 2

Total score was obtained simply by addition of scores on these two sub-scales, and might range from 0–4.

Results

Distribution of dependence scores. 44 per cent gave dependence score 0, 21 per cent score 1 or 2, 33 per cent score 3 or 4 (not classified 2 per cent), with n = 188. Analysis was then made of relationship between dependence score and factors which are grouped sequentially under the headings: (a) crime, (b) the drinking problem, (c) social stability.

For all analyses the sample size (n) employed in the particular cross-tabulation will be indicated; because of unsatisfactory completion of forms, etc., this number is in all instances slightly below the base 188.

Drinking and crime. Table 8.1 presents a summary of relationships between dependence scores and aspects of criminality.

There is a consistent tendency for stepwise differences with increased dependence score. In this and similar summary tables the notation will be used of indicating significance of difference between proportions (x^2 on raw scores), of entries in adjacent columns thus: 0 not significant; – P < .05; = P < .01

Drink, a problem now. There is a significant stepwise increased likelihood of such admission with increased dependence score.

Average daily intake of beer or cider. Taking ten pints as the cut-off, a score of 1, 2 significantly differentiates subjects from those scoring 0, while the 1, 2

Table 8.1
Drinking and crime

Question	0	Sig.	1,2	Sig.	3,4
Present offence a drunkenness offence	11 $(\frac{9}{83})$	=	43 $(\frac{17}{40})$	–	63 $(\frac{39}{62})$
6+ arrests for drunkenness	10 $(\frac{8}{83})$	=	41 $(\frac{16}{39})$	=	82 $(\frac{51}{62})$
11+ times in prison	5 $(\frac{3}{66})$	=	29 $(\frac{10}{35})$	0	44 $(\frac{24}{54})$
Sentence – 4 weeks	29 $(\frac{24}{82})$	=	58 $(\frac{23}{40})$	0	73 $(\frac{45}{62})$
Drinking immediately before arrest	41 $(\frac{34}{83})$	=	85 $(\frac{34}{40})$	=	95 $(\frac{59}{62})$
Drunk at time of offence	27 $(\frac{22}{81})$	=	71 $(\frac{27}{38})$	0	83 $(\frac{50}{60})$
Amnesia related to present offence	1 $(\frac{1}{81})$	0	8 $(\frac{3}{40})$	=	29 $(\frac{18}{62})$
All criminal charges due to drink	20 $(\frac{15}{76})$	–	40 $(\frac{16}{40})$	0	56 $(\frac{35}{62})$

% in grouped dependence categories answering affirmatively to questions in left hand column, raw scores in brackets.

For notation of significance levels see text.

subjects are here almost identical with those scoring 3, 4. Further analysis does however show that subjects scoring 3, 4 are more likely to be found in the upper tail of those drinking 19 pints or more (21/59, 36 per cent of 3, 4: 7/40, 18 per cent of 1, 2: 4/83, 5 per cent of 0 scoring subjects). The correlation between pints on average day and dependence score is 0.330.

Experience of amnesia due to drinking. There is a significant stepwise relationship between increasing dependence score and increasing likelihood of experience of amnesia 'often'.

Admission for hospital inpatient treatment of alcoholism. Table 8.2 shows that subjects with a score of 0 are extremely unlikely (2 per cent) to have

Table 8.2
The drinking problem

Question	% in grouped dependence categories answering affirmatively, raw scores in brackets.				
	0	Sig.	1,2	Sig.	3,4
Drink, a problem now	10 $(\frac{8}{83})$	=	44 $(\frac{17}{39})$	=	84 $(\frac{52}{62})$
Average daily intake greater than 10 pints beer or cider	18 $(\frac{15}{83})$	=	65 $(\frac{26}{40})$	0	66 $(\frac{39}{59})$
Experience of amnesia 'often'	10 $(\frac{8}{83})$	=	43 $(\frac{17}{40})$	=	77 $(\frac{48}{62})$
Hospital in-patient care for alcoholism ever	2 $(\frac{2}{83})$	0	3 $(\frac{1}{40})$	=	45 $(\frac{28}{62})$

For notation of significance levels see text.

received inpatient treatment for alcoholism, and those with 1, 2 dependence scores closely resemble them (3 per cent) – in this population a moderate dependence score does not lead to treatment. These two groups (0 and 1, 2) stand in significant contrast to those with a 3, 4 score, where 45 per cent have received treatment.

Ever in Camberwell Reception Centre. The centre referred to is a large shelter for homeless men in South London, run by the Department of Health and Social Security, (Edwards et al., 1968). Table 8.3 shows a significant stepwise increase in likelihood of having ever been in the centre with increased dependence score.

Longest at one address during the previous six months. Here the significant contrast is between, on the one hand those scoring 0 and on the other, those scoring either 1, 2 or 3, 4. Correlation between the two variables is – 0.479.

Months in last job. Table 8.3 shows a consistent trend for job instability to be associated with higher dependence scores but the findings do not reach a level of significance – those with a dependence score of 3, 4 had a more than 50 per cent chance of only short employment.

Discussion

1 *Methodological limitations.* The very special nature of the sample has

Table 8.3
Social stability

Question	% in grouped dependence categories answering affirmatively, raw scores in brackets.				
	0	Sig.	1,2	Sig.	3,4
Ever in Camberwell Reception Centre	28 $(\frac{23}{82})$	–	48 $(\frac{19}{40})$	=	79 $(\frac{49}{62})$
Longest residence at one address during previous 6 months, 4 or less weeks	7 $(\frac{5}{76})$	=	30 $(\frac{11}{37})$	0	34 $(\frac{18}{53})$
Period in last job less than 1 month	19 $(\frac{15}{80})$	0	33 $(\frac{13}{40})$	0	52 $(\frac{27}{53})$

For notation of significance levels see text.

already been stressed. The scale of dependence developed here is very crude. Class and personality factors were not controlled, and although this population is relatively homogenous for class, the same assumption cannot be made for personality. Reliability and validity are undetermined; response set may have affected replies to unknown degree.

2 *Implications for the understanding of alcoholism.* The hypothesis which receives some very provisional support from present findings is that the social consequences to the individual of his abnormal drinking may be determined by (among other things) the intensity of a specific core pathology – the intensity of *dependence*. The 'other things' – the pathoplastic factors – must include class and personality (Chandler et al., 1971), and no doubt other variables besides. The weighting and the nature of the interaction of these variables is unknown, and must depend on the particular outcome variable. In mathematical terms, the model is no more precise than:

Outcomes = f (dependence, personality, class . . .)

Other than its introduction of quantifiable dependence, such an equation is so all-embracing as to be neither contentious nor particularly heuristic – the only notion contained in it which is other than common and accepted wisdom is the postulate that *degree of dependence* is of predictive value.

3 *Implications for research.* The predictive value of the present very rough

and ready method of scoring dependence suggests a number of leads for research.

(a) *Construction of a scientifically more satisfactory scale.* A more finely discriminative scale is needed, with both reliability and validity determined.

(b) *Progression and regression of dependence.* If dependence can be accurately measured change in intensity over time could be the subject of longitudinal study. Are there particular points on the curve which represent growth of dependence over time, at which growth is likely suddenly to accelerate – is what is clinically recognised as alcoholism a point of inflection on such a curve? Is growth after a certain point exponential? Are there sections of the curve at which regression, 'forgetting' in learning terms, 'return to normal drinking' in clinical terms (Davies, 1962), is likely, and other sections where such happenings do not occur? Is drinking after a period of abstinence followed by more or less rapid re-establishment of a high degree of dependence contingent on the degree of dependence previously achieved – is something observable akin to a reminiscence effect?

(c) *Animal experiment.* The idea of dependence being quantifiable might be fruitful in advancing animal work.

4 *Implications for policy.* A simple questionnaire allows identification of a group of men who form a not inconsiderable proportion of the inmates of a short term recidivist prison. These men are identified as suffering from alcohol dependence and the degree of this dependence is predictive of certain aspects of their criminal behaviour. Even moderate dependence is a condition far from benign in its social implications.

Those subjects who score 1, 2 show increased likelihood of varieties of social disability; sadly, they are at present almost exempt from likelihood of receiving treatment.

8.2 Prevalence of drinking problems among short term and long term recidivist prisoners

The purpose of this investigation was to obtain a number of prevalence estimates on the basis of different definitions of pathology, with an examination as to how the seemingly diverse estimates might logically be reconciled. The population comprised the two contrasting groups of operationally defined short term and long term prisoners, with the expectation that considerable prevalence differences might be shown up between these two groups.

Results

Throughout this report the abbreviations LT and ST will indicate the total long term (one year or longer) sentence group and short term (less than three months) sentence group respectively. ST drunk will refer to short term men who are currently in prison because of a drunkenness offence, while ST non-drunk refers to the remainder of the short term group.

Dependence score distributions. Table 8.4 shows the distribution of subjects between dependence score categories. On the basis of this analysis it can be said that:

(i)   LT, and ST non-drunk, do not differ significantly: the percentages with 0 scores are close, as are the percentages with DS 1, 2; while the percentages with DS 3, 4 (11 v 19 per cent) differ a little more.

(ii)   The ST drunk group differ significantly both from the LT and ST non-drunk (P < 0.01 in either instance with x^2 testing of subjects scoring DS 0, versus those scoring DS 1 or more). The major difference lies, however, not in the DS 1, 2 category but in the DS 3, 4 category percentage – it is in the high proportion of subjects with major degree of dependence that the ST drunk group contrasts with the other two prisoner groups.

Table 8.4
Dependence score distributions

	Dependence score categories: raw percentage			
	n	0	1,2	3,4
Long term, total	312	66	23	11
Short term, total	285	45	22	33
ST non-drunks	120	62	19	19
ST drunks	65	14	26	60

Pointers to heavy or abnormal drinking, and mean DS. Table 8.5 summarises answers to a range of questions and gives mean dependence scores for subgroups answering positively or negatively to each of these questions.

(i)   The ST drunk group is in every instance extreme as regards percentage report.

(ii)   ST non-drunk group on all pointers shows a higher percentage incidence than does LT, but according to the particular item the degree of difference varies considerably and may be trivial or large.

(iii)   Inspection of the mean dependence scores gives some guide as to which items are more strongly related to drinking pathology.

Table 8.5

Pointers to abnormal drinking and mean dependence scores. Note that in some instances the numbers involved are small.

			Long term	Short term: total	Short term: non-drunk	Short term: drunk
Drink, a problem now:		% total	16	43	26	77
	Mean DS	Yes	2.5	3.0	2.7	3.2
		No	0.4	0.6	0.5	1.5
Daily alcohol		% total	14	49	36	73
10 pints beer:	Mean DS	Yes	2.0	2.4	1.7	3.1
		No	0.6	0.9	0.7	1.9
Amnesia once/twice:		% total	18	40	26	65
	Mean DS	Yes	2.6	3.1	2.7	3.3
		No	0.4	0.8	0.5	1.9
Inpatient for alcoholism		% total	03	17	07	35
ever:	Mean DS	Yes	3.4	3.6	3.4	3.7
		No	0.7	1.3	0.9	2.3

Drinking and criminal involvement. Information on relation between drinking and criminal involvement is summarised in Table 8.6; mean dependence score comparisons between sub-groups answering 'yes' or 'no' again give an indication as to the degree to which an item is related to dependence.

(i) Items a, b, c of Table 8.6 may be taken as indicating intoxication of progressively severe degree; the difference between LT, ST non-drunk and ST drunk is consistent.

(ii) Neither drinking for Dutch courage, nor crime directed toward acquisition of money for drink, are common.

(iii) A history of one of more drunkenness arrests (item f) shows in each prisoner group an association with raised DS score, while with a history of 6+ arrests (item g) this relationship is more strongly marked. A history of 6+ drunkenness offences differentiates sharply between LT (6 per cent) and ST drunk (83 per cent), with ST non-drunk giving an intermediate 18 per cent.

58

Table 8.6
Drinking and criminal involvement and mean dependence scores

			Long term	Short term: total	Short term: non-drunk	Short term: drunk
a. Drinking immediately before offence:		% total	41	69	52	100
	Mean DS	Yes	1.4	2.3	1.7	2.8
		No	0.3	0.4	0.4	–
b. Drunk at time of present offence:		% total	14	56	34	95
	Mean DS	Yes	2.1	2.4	2.0	2.7
		No	0.5	0.8	0.7	3.7
c. Amnesia for present offence:		% total	04	12	05	25
	Mean DS	Yes	2.5	3.4	3.0	3.6
		No	0.7	1.5	1.0	2.6
d. Drank for courage to commit present offence:		% total	04	02	03	02
	Mean DS	Yes	1.5	3.0	2.7	4.0
		No	0.8	1.7	1.0	2.8
e. Present offence acquisitive for money to drink:		% total	06	06	08	02
	Mean DS	Yes	2.3	1.8	1.8	2.0
		No	0.7	1.7	1.0	2.9
f. 1 or more arrests for drunkenness:		% total	24	64	45	100
	Mean DS	Yes	1.7	2.5	2.1	2.8
		No	0.5	0.3	0.2	
g. 6 or more arrests for drunkenness:		% total	06	41	18	83
	Mean DS	Yes	2.7	3.1	3.1	3.1
		No	0.7	0.7	0.6	1.6

1 *Questions of prevalence.* The prevalence of abnormal drinking in a prison or in any other population must be dependent on the chosen definition. In the long term prisoner group, for instance, if the criterion of abnormal drinking is six or more arrests for drunkenness, prevalence is 6 per cent; report of severe dependence (DS 3, 4) gives 11 per cent; drunkenness at time of offence 14 per cent: the subject's own perception of drink being a problem gives 16 per cent prevalence; a history or one or more drunkenness arrests gives 24 per cent; some evidence of dependence (DS 1–4) makes the figure 34 per cent; report of drinking immediately before arrest gives a 41 per cent prevalence. How, in logic, is a decision made as to which index provides the most 'correct' prevalence estimate?

To make sense of this perplexing state of affairs one has to turn back from examination of the answers to a closer scrutiny of the actual questioning. Rather than all the different questions constituting so many absolute alternatives, they can be grouped into three types: (a) prevalence of a defined syndrome, (b) levels of alcohol consumption and (c) prevalence of adverse consequences of drinking.

(a) *Prevalence of a defined syndrome.* If there were universal agreement as to the existence of a disease entity called 'alcoholism', and if there were then unequivocal and clearly recognisable symptoms of that disease, the epidemiologists' task would be as simple as counting cases of measles. Such, unfortunately, is generally not the case; there are conflicting theories as to what constitutes alcoholism and how that condition is to be differentiated from heavy drinking; the criteria for definition which these theories would propose are often both vague and subtle – for example, loss of control – and not readily susceptible to the strict operational definition required for survey purposes.

Dependence scores seek to operationalise the concept of alcohol dependence (alcohol addiction) as disorder of learning. Much more work is needed before the validity of this approach can be determined. What a dependence score aims to measure is a core pathology rather than the (symptomatic) social, physical, or mental consequences which result from that pathology – it asks about measles rather than about time missed from school. The model proposes that any statement on prevalence must differentiate between degrees of the syndrome's severity and, in simple terms, hopes to provide an estimate of subjects who are 'moderately addicted' and 'very addicted'.

(b) *Alcohol consumption.* Ten pints is a quite arbitrary cut off point, and data on drinking quantity – or drinking frequency – is to be seen more as an added hint regarding the type of drinking population we are dealing with, than as a precise or very useful prevalence measure.

(c) *Prevalence of adverse consequences of drinking.* Adverse consequences may occur from drinking when the subject is not alcohol dependent – not all drunkenness or drunken mishaps are symptomatic of actual dependence on the drug. One way of estimating the prevalence of persons who are experiencing troubles due to drinking is to ask a very general question either of an independent informant or of the subject himself; whether informant or subject is the witness, it is only their perception of the matter which is being recorded, and such perception may for many reasons be vulnerable to denial or distortion. The reality of denial is suggested by 23 per cent of men who are at present imprisoned on a drunkenness charge, denying that drink is a problem.

Another way in which 'problem' drinkers may be enumerated is, rather than using the holistic approach, to make inquiry as to the possible occurrence of a whole range of specific adverse events which the subject perceives as having been caused by his drinking (Edwards et al., 1972). One such item is the occurrence of alcoholic amnesias. Figures from the present survey (Table 8.4) with 18, 26, and 65 per cent report of occurrence 'more than once or twice' for LT, ST non-drunk and ST drunk, respectively, are percentages not very different from those that come from the holistic questioning on 'drink, now a problem'.

Bringing together these various lines of evidence, they may thus be seen to complement rather than contradict each other. For the three prisoner groups, matters may be summarised thus:

(i) Long term. Of the three groups, this population shows – whatever the chosen measure – the lowest prevalence of drinking pathology. About one man in ten (11 per cent) admits to symptoms which suggest likelihood of severe alcohol dependence, with approximately twice as many (23 per cent) giving indications suggestive of more mild dependence; such mild dependence is not at all certainly related to subjective awareness of 'a problem'. The 14 per cent of subjects drinking more than 10 pints a day suggests that we are dealing with an abnormally heavy drinking population. Sixteen per cent admit to subjective awareness of drink being a problem now; the rates given for frequent amnesia and for drunkenness arrest suggest that this figure might perhaps have to be corrected somewhat upwards for an estimate of the percentage whose lives are being more or less troubled by their drinking.

(ii) Short term non-drunk. All indicators suggest that for drinking pathology this is the intermediate group, with perhaps about two out of ten (19 per cent) severely alcohol dependent and the same proportion more mildly dependent – the rate of heavy drinking (36 > 10 pints a day) is much in excess of that found among the long term men. Twenty-six per cent admit to drink now being a problem, a figure agreeing with frequent amnesia, but much below that for drunkenness arrest (45 per cent).

(iii)   Short term drunk. This is on all criteria the most troubled group – six out of ten (60 per cent) admit to symptoms suggestive of severe alcohol dependence and three out of ten (26 per cent) to mild dependence; heavy drinking is the norm (73 > 10 pints per day) and eight out of ten (77 per cent) admit to drink now being a problem; report of amnesias (65 > twice) and, of course, of drunkenness arrest (100 per cent), confirm the extent of disturbance.

2   *Implications for policy.* The results suggest the need for the feasibly controlled experiment which would determine the effect of treatment on criminal recidivism of prisoners with defined drinking pathology. That proper after-care is, of course, of some utility with the chronic drunkenness offender seems, however, very likely from the evidence already presented by Cook et al. (1968), and in any well-conceived therapeutic experiment 'therapy' should mean both care and after-care.

9 The drunk in court: survey of drunkenness offenders from two London courts*

DENIS GATH, CELIA HENSMAN, ANN HAWKER, MICHAEL KELLY and GRIFFITH EDWARDS

Summary

One hundred and fifty-one drunkenness offenders were interviewed immediately after appearance before the magistrate: the survey was conducted in two Metropolitan (London) courts: one was in an area frequented by vagrants and the other in a more mixed suburb. The majority of those interviewed had a serious drinking problem and 50 per cent showed evidence of well established alcohol dependence. Gross social isolation was the rule. The bearing of these findings on the planning of apt helping services is discussed.

Introduction

The problem of society's response to the drunkenness offender is at present much under discussion. A Home Office working party was at the time of this study reviewing the question of 'the treatment, within the penal system, of persons who habitually commit offences involving drunkenness'. [1] Its deliberations were given urgency by Section 91 of the Criminal Justice Act, 1967 (Great Britain Laws Statutes, 1968) which proposes that imprisonment for a 'drunk and disorderly' offence be abolished as soon as alternative accommodation is available for the care and treatment of offenders. The first International Congress on the Drunkenness Offence was held in London in May 1968 (Cook et al., 1969). Several speakers there reported a move in other European countries and the USA to treat the public inebriate as a sick person and to exclude him entirely from the courts and from the criminal process.

Every year in England and Wales there are upwards of 75,000 convictions for drunkenness with or without 'aggravations', a number which makes heavy demands on the resources of the police and courts. Yet little is known about

---

* A slightly shortened version of a paper of the same title originally appearing in the *British Medical Journal,* vol. 4, 1968, pp. 808–11.

the kind of person the drunkenness offender is, and the impact on him of arrest and conviction is little understood. The official statistics are limited to an analysis of drunkenness offences by geographical regions, and by sex and age of offenders (Home Office, 1968). Offences of this kind are not recorded centrally, and there is no indication of what proportion of them are caused by habitual offenders and what proportion by 'once only' offenders. Prison records are not helpful here, there being no reason to suppose that inebriates in prison are representative of drunkenness offenders as a whole. Previous surveys in the court setting have been carried out in London (Parr, 1962), Rochester, USA (Zax et al., 1964), and Toronto (Giffen, 1966–8); these studies were of limited scope, as they did not include interviews with offenders but were based on scrutiny of court records, from which only simple demographic data can be drawn.

An editorial in the *British Medical Journal* (1968) drew attention to the dearth of research information concerning the kinds of people who are arrested for drunkenness, and emphasised that 'the proportion of drunkenness offenders who are casual roisterers as opposed to people with serious drinking problems or sufferers from alcohol dependence remains obscure'. The answer to this question is relevant to any discussion regarding reform of the law and the design of therapeutic alternatives to fine or imprisonment: the aim of the present investigation was to obtain information bearing directly on this question. More specifically, the aim was to interview a sample of men appearing in London courts on drunkenness charges, in order to study their social and psychological characteristics and to determine (1) what proportion showed evidence of chemical dependence on alcohol, and (2) what proportion were suffering from social breakdown and isolation.

Method

Ideally, sampling would have been carried out at all the 16 Metropolitan magistrates' courts, but in the course of extensive inquiries at these courts it became clear that this was impracticable for several reasons, such as lack of interviewing space.

Two courts were therefore selected as being representative of contrasting types of area, the one (court A) in a poor and run-down quarter where vagrants tend to congregate, the other (court B) in a mixed working class and middle class residential area. Drunkenness offenders were interviewed by a psychiatrist (DG, GE, MK) or by a research assistant (CH, AH) who had previous experience in alcoholism studies. A semi-structured interviewing schedule was used which consisted of 80 questions and took 20 to 30 minutes to complete. In pre-pilot work, interviews were tape-recorded and subsequently discussed by the investigators in a group, so that uniformity of interviewing techniques and precise agreement on criteria were achieved. A six-week pilot study consisting of 47 interviews was then carried out in the two courts and the schedule revised.

The definitive study ran from 1 September 1967 to 16 January 1968 and consisted of 151 interviews, of which 84 were at court A and 67 at court B. Interviewing was carried out every Monday, Wednesday, Friday, and Saturday, using a simple fortnightly rota so that visits to the two courts were evenly distributed over the days of the week. Offenders were seen immediately after appearing before the magistrates, and participation was voluntary. Only male subjects charged with a drunkenness offence were included in the survey; motoring and other drink-associated offences were excluded.

The sampling procedure was to interview the first two offenders passing through the court each day, and as many of the rest as time permitted. No bias was introduced by this procedure, because the order of appearance in court is determined fortuitously by the varying order in which offenders arrive from various police stations. Supporting evidence that the sample was not biased was afforded by basic data which were collected on the total population of male drunkenness offenders, both interviewed and not-interviewed, passing through the two courts during the survey period.

Co-operation of interviewees.

Less than five per cent of men refused to participate in this survey, and 90 per cent of those who complied were rated as 'fully co-operative'.

Results

Of the 151 men in the total sample, 70 per cent had been charged with being drunk, 22 per cent with being drunk and disorderly, and the remaining 8 per cent with miscellaneous charges such as drunk and indecent, etc. Two-thirds of the total sample had been remanded in custody, while one-third had been allowed bail.

The between-court analyses showed that the great majority of results were similar at the two courts; findings will not therefore be routinely presented for the courts separately, the results being similar unless otherwise stated.

1   *Demographic data*

The age range of the total sample (n = 151) was 18–79, the mean age at court B, 39.4 years, being significantly lower than at court A, 44.0 years (P < 0.05). There was a preponderance of men from the lower social classes relative to

65

the country as a whole, as determined by the Registrar General's classification of occupational status: classes I and II two per cent, class III 27 per cent, class IV 18 per cent, class V 48 per cent, not classifiable five per cent. The offender's country of birth was given as England 36 per cent, Southern Ireland 34 per cent, Scotland 13 per cent, Northern Ireland four per cent, Wales three per cent, coloured two per cent, other eight per cent. There was an excess of those reared in the Catholic faith; Roman Catholic 58 per cent, Established Church 33 per cent, Nonconformist four per cent, Jewish nil, other five per cent. Of the total sample 56 per cent had never married; only 17 per cent were living with their wives; 11 per cent were divorced or legally separated, while 11 per cent had a non-legal separation; three per cent were widowed; two per cent admitted co-habiting.

2   Circumstances of arrest

In response to inquiry about the circumstances of the drinking that led to arrest, nine per cent of the total sample named a celebration or special social event such as an anniversary, party, or club meeting; two per cent stated that they were seeking consolation after a traumatic event such as a bereavement or loss of job; while 17 per cent said they were drinking because it was pay-day. The great majority (70 per cent) could give no special reason for drinking, or reported simply that they were bored or lonely. Of the offenders 37 per cent had been entirely alone while drinking; 30 per cent had consumed no food during the 24 hours before arrest; and six per cent admitted drinking methylated spirits immediately before arrest.

3   Previous drunkenness and criminal involvement

In the 12 months preceding this arrest 21 per cent of the sample had been arrested for drunkenness once or twice, ten per cent from three to five times, ten per cent from six to ten times; six per cent from 11 to 25 times, and four per cent over 25 times − that is to say, 51 per cent had been arrested on at least one previous occasion during the past 12 months; and 24 per cent admitted to one or more arrests during the four preceding weeks. At some time 26 per cent had been charged with 'property offences', 20 per cent with other petty offences, and nine per cent with offences of violence. Most of these charges appeared to be drink-related. Forty-five per cent had been in prison at least once, and 24 per cent had been on probation at some time.

4   Beverage choice

The majority of this sample were habitual beer drinkers, but 18 per cent admitted that rough cider or cheap wine was their customary drink.

Inquiry was made about the subject's experience of alcoholic amnesias and of symptoms usually taken as indicative of chemical dependence, such as morning shakes, morning relief drinking, 'loss of control,' and hallucinatory experiences.

Amnesias for the night before had been experienced at some time by 79 per cent of subjects, day-time amnesias by 27 per cent, and amnesias lasting at least 24 hours by 13 per cent. Forty-six per cent reported having had an alcoholic fugue from which they had 'woken up' in a strange part of the town or a distant city with no recollection of how they had journeyed there – an occurrence which we have termed the 'journey syndrome'.

Morning shakes had been experienced by 62 per cent of the total sample; 50 per cent reported morning relief drinking, and half of these (25 per cent of the total) admitted this was habitual. On detailed questioning 49 per cent of subjects had clearly experienced 'loss of control' over their drinking – five per cent within the last year only, 24 per cent for one to five years, and 20 per cent for a period over five years.

Seventeen per cent of subjects were found to have suffered from delirium tremens at one time or another, as determined strictly by the criteria outlined by Victor and Adams (1953). The syndrome of alcoholic hallucinosis, defined equally rigorously, was identified in seven per cent of the sample, while a further 23 per cent reported having experienced transient visual or auditory hallucinations.

In every case an attempt was made to assess the severity of the subject's drinking problem by detailed questioning about the pattern of his drinking habits, including his drinking milieu, beverage choice, amount consumed, and frequency and times of day of drinking. Information was also sought concerning social and medical damage resulting from drinking. Thirty-two per cent had pawned and 24 per cent admitted begging or stealing to raise money for drinking. Twenty-two per cent had been barred from hostels, 32 per cent had had a serious accident and 26 per cent a head injury resulting in unconsciousness, 16 per cent had suffered from peptic ulceration, and eight per cent indicated that they had attempted suicide at some time.

On the basis of all the above information, at the completion of each interview the investigators attempted to allocate the subject to one of the five categories of alcoholism defined by Jellinek (1960). Table 9.1 shows that 24 per cent of the total sample were not considered to have a serious drinking problem; 26 per cent were judged to have a serious problem without being chemically dependent on alcohol (alpha alcoholism); while 50 per cent were showing clear-cut evidence of chemical dependence (gamma, delta, or epsilon), and could therefore be designated 'alcoholics' or 'alcohol addicts', however broadly or narrowly these terms might be defined.

Table 9.1

Classification of offenders by Jellinek typology

Jellinek category	Total sample (n=151) %	Court A (n=84) %	Court B (n=67) %
'No problem'	24	17	32
Alpha	26	25	27
Beta	–	–	–
Gamma	45	50	39
Delta	1	1	2
Epsilon	4	7	–
	100	100	100

Table 9.2 shows the relation between certain factors and classification in the gamma-delta-epsilon as opposed to the alpha or no problem categories. A x^2 test on the distribution of each of the items shows significant differences at the levels indicated.

The contributions of the individual cells to the overall x^2 value indicate that in respect of factors 1, 4, 5 and 6 (no fixed abode, usually drinking rough cider or cheap wine, more than ten arrests for drunkenness in the past 12 months, and regular use of drugs) the alpha and no problem groups resemble one another fairly closely. However, in factor 2 (divorced or separated) the alpha resembles more closely the gamma-delta-epsilon category, and in factor 3 (Irish origin) the three groups are all dissimilar.

6 Social isolation

The majority of offenders were found to be grossly lacking in social support. An indication of this was given by their accommodation at the time of arrest – as shown in Table 9.3, only 42 per cent had accommodation of their own, in the sense of a house, flat, or furnished room. As mentioned above, only 17 per cent of the total were married and living with their spouse.

Table 9.2
Relation of certain social factors to classification of offenders by Jellinek typology

		No problem (n=34) %	Alpha (n=39) %	Gamma, delta, epsilon (n=76) %	χ^2 level	Probability level
1	No fixed abode	9	10	33	12.0	<0.005
2	Divorced or separated	3	26	31	10.2	<0.01
3	Irish by birth	24	33	48	6.2	<0.05
4	Usual drink: rough cider/ cheap wine	6	8	30	12.3	<0.005
5	More than 10 arrests for drunkenness in past 12 months	0	0	15	11.4	<0.005
6	Drugs used regularly at some time	6	3	19	7.7	<0.025

Of those who had previously been married (27 per cent), very few (15 per cent of the subgroup) had any contact with their children or former wife during the preceding 12 months, while 55 per cent of the total sample had no contact with their parents or siblings in that period. Forty per cent of the offenders had not attended a cinema, dance, church, or other social function in the preceding five years. Less than ten per cent belonged to a club, union, or similar organisation. Forty-two per cent had slept in a reception centre and 51 per cent had slept rough at times. The occupational history of these offenders showed marked instability: at the time of arrest 40 per cent were unemployed, while of the employed half had been in their current job for under three months and only a quarter for more than a year. Fifty per cent had held more than five jobs in five years. There was a significantly higher (P < 0.01) proportion of offenders in social class V when classified according to their present or most recent job status as against their 'best job ever'.

7   Court disposal for current offences

This is shown in Table 9.4. The distribution of disposals does not differ significantly from that of the total population of both courts during the study period.

Table 9.3
Offenders' accommodation at time of arrest

	Total (n=151) %	Court A (n=84) %	Court B (n=67) %
Own accommodation	42	25	64
Ordinary hostel	23	36	7
No fixed abode	21	23	19
Old people's home	3	4	3
Alcoholic hostel	3	1	5
Just discharged from prison	3	6	–
Reception centre	2	4	–
Other	3	1	2
	100	100	100

Table 9.4
Court disposal for offences

Sentence	%
Discharge: absolute or conditional	5
'10s. or one day'	23
Fine paid	42
Fine with time to pay*	24
Prison or remand	6
	100

* Some of these men were later sent to prison because of failure to pay their fines within the stated time.

8 Previous treatment for alcoholism

Past treatments which the offenders reported having received were: psychiatric treatment for alcoholism, 19 per cent; admission to an alcoholics' hostel, 12 per cent; regular attendance at Alcoholics Anonymous meetings, eight per cent.

9   *Professed willingness to accept help*

The subjects' willingness to accept future help was briefly assessed, but with no effort at persuasion or detailed explanation. Table 9.5 shows the proportions in the Jellinek alpha-no-problem category as against the gamma-delta-epsilon category who said they would definitely be willing to accept medical or social help. A χ^2 test showed that the differences were significant at the 0.1 per cent level.

Table 9.5
Subjects' attitude to medical or social help by Jellinek classification

	No problem, alpha (n=73) %	Gamma, delta, epsilon (n=76) %	χ^2 (with Yates's correction)	Probability
Medical help	5	38	21.2	<0.001
Social help	1	26	17.1	<0.001

Discussion

In discussing the implications of this survey it is necessary to consider how far the populations of these two courts are representative of the country in general. This cannot be determined without further studies in other localities, but two factors suggest that the results may be widely applicable.

First, the drunkenness offence is largely a big-city problem, and to this extent it is reasonable to suppose that the results provide a typical picture of the national situation. Secondly, the two courts were selected as being representative of areas with different socio-economic characteristics in the expectation that the results would disclose the main differences between the kinds of drunkenness offender in a run-down city area and those in a stable residential area. To some extent such differences were found, as, for example, in the degrees of 'rootlessness' of the two offender populations (Table 9.3). In most respects, however, it is the similarity of the findings at the two courts which calls for comment. It was found, for example, that there were certain between-court differences in types of drinking problem (Table 9.1), and yet the proportions of men showing evidence of chemical dependence were of similar magnitude at the two courts.

There was no check on the reliability of data collected in the survey, and generalisations based on the responses of drunkenness offenders should be made with caution. However, there are several reasons for supposing that the subjects were not motivated to be other than truthful. Interviews were conducted after the court hearing had taken place, and the interviewers emphasised that they were engaged on medical research rather than an 'official' inquiry. The internal consistency of the results also suggests their accuracy. In a previous inquiry (Edwards et al., 1966b) responses given by Skid Row alcoholics were found to tally closely with official criminal and hospital records. Furthermore, studies in Toronto (Giffen, 1966–8) have suggested that in surveys of this kind any distortion tends towards an underestimate rather than an overestimate of the extent and severity of pathological drinking and social disruption.

The picture which emerges from this survey is therefore at least an approximate answer to the question posed by the *British Medical Journal* (1968) cited above. 'Casual roisterers' formed a small proportion – slightly less than a quarter – of the sample of drunkenness offenders; men with a serious drinking problem which had not advanced to addiction formed a quarter, while as many as one-half showed evidence of chemical dependence on alcohol. The results further showed that a large proportion of the men were labouring under a gross degree of social breakdown and isolation.

What light does the survey throw on existing methods of treating the public drunk? Thirty per cent stated that they had been arrested three or more times in the preceding 12 months, while only 19 per cent reported having had psychiatric treatment for alcoholism, and a mere 12 per cent had found their way into an alcoholism rehabilitation centre. In most cases the courts are being asked to deal with problems for which judicial processes are inappropriate. If the inference is made that some other method of treatment is called for, and that such men should be cast in the sick role rather than the criminal role, it does not follow that conventional hospital treatment will meet their needs. This is because, after a period of hospital treatment, these men must return to a world in which demonstrably they lack the social skills to survive, having lost or never having possessed such skills.

If present methods of treatment are unsuitable or inadequate, what are the implications of the survey for planning future measures? The guide is probably given by the gross social isolation found in the bulk of the offenders. Their needs are most likely to be met by treating this social isolation in providing a supportive environment (Myerson, 1953) or a therapeutic community which can teach them new skills (Edwards et al., 1966a). At present special hostels for chronic alcoholics are being tried out in London (Cook et al., 1968), and these would seem to be the most promising way of providing the 'suitable accommodation' envisaged by the Criminal Justice Act (Great Britain, 1968). Such hostels might form part of an integrated rehabilitation service which could include a 'shop front' counselling centre and a short-term detoxication centre (Pittman, 1968).

Such a programme inevitably raises the question of the subject's motivation. That 22 per cent of offenders stated they would accept immediate medical or social treatment suggests a sizable service need. As for the remainder, it would be unjustifiable to dismiss them as 'unmotivated' in the absence of services designed to meet their special needs. It has been shown that such men can be responsive to special methods of hostel treatment if these methods are implemented with patience and skill (Cook et al., 1968). The challenge should be accepted of designing services accurately to meet these special needs, following which unmotivated men may well become motivated towards further treatment.

There are grounds, too, for proposing that other measures are required for the casual roisterer. In the popular stereotype the roisterer is usually taken as a figure of fun, but he may well be the alcohol addict of the future. A first incident of public drunkenness may presage serious trouble ahead. Every chronic drunk was once a first offender, and when a man comes up for the first time before the magistrates this may indeed be the live opportunity for early detection of a problem and for an early offer of help.

Notes

[1] Its findings appeared as the Home Office Report on *Habitual Drunken Offenders* (1971): HMSO, London.

10   Occupation as a possible cause of alcoholism*

T. A. SPRATLEY

Summary

Logical problems which beset the attempt to infer from occupation correlation an occupational causation of alcoholism are considered. Unstructured pre-pilot interviews were conducted with subjects working in a variety of supposedly drink-exposed occupations and six possible factors related to drink exposure identified. A questionnaire was then administered to 390 alcoholics. Occupational pressure may be less important than commonsense would propose.

Review was first made of previously published evidence for the importance of occupation factors in the genesis of alcoholism. There is a common belief that any occupation which is concerned with manufacture, distribution or sale of liquor, carries a high risk of alcoholism, and British figures are quoted to show a cirrhosis mortality rate among publicans which is nine times the expected level. Among other groups classically said to be at risk are salesmen, people in entertainment and communication professions, e.g., actors, musicians, journalists, merchant seamen, members of the regular Armed Forces; company directors and business managers, and a miscellaneous group including butchers and dock labourers.

Detailed analysis is then made of the logical problems which beset any attempt to infer from occupational correlation an occupational causality. Reference is made to general criteria put forward by Bradford Hill (1965) as serving to support the causality of the relationship between two associated variables. Special factors are then identified as influencing the actual number of alcoholics (however defined and enumerated), who will be found at any one time in a survey of any given occupational group:

1   Factors causal of increased prevalence:
(a)   the true alcoholism-generating influence of that occupation;
(b)   pre-selection into that occupation of alcoholics and people pre-disposed to become alcoholics;

---

* Synopsis of an unpublished dissertation of the same title by T. A. Spratley which was submitted successfully in 1969 to the University of London in part fulfilment of requirements for the degree of M. Phil.

(c)   secondary selection: certain occupations are transitional ones from which people normally move on to better jobs; those who remain might be handicapped individuals, who could be pre-disposed to alcoholism.

2   Factors causal of decreased prevalence:

(a)   pre-selection into the occupation of individuals who are extremely stable and non-predisposed to alcoholism;

(b)   secondary selection out of that occupation of alcoholics and pre-disposed alcoholics.

The potential snares and pitfalls which may trip up any too simplistic interpretation of an observed relationship are illustrated by considering the occupation of airline pilots. A survey of pilots might be expected to show a very low prevalence of alcoholism indeed; the job is hardly compatible with the intoxicated state. Could it, therefore, be concluded that this particular occupation is protective against alcoholism? Exactly the contrary might theoretically be the case: the stresses and strains of the job might be highly alcoholism-inducing, but because men who developed even an early drinking problem would leave the profession, the occupation prevalence rate would be low.

A model is developed which on the basis of the usual interactional (multi-causal) theory of the genesis of alcoholism should allow logical testing of the contribution of 'factor X'. The assumptions inherent to the model are spelled out in detail, and situations in which the validity of assumption might break down are identified.

With the theoretical base thus established, some original survey work is reported. This was in pre-pilot, pilot and definitive phases and the particular style of investigation owes much to the teachings of A. N. Oppenheim (1966).

In the pre-pilot work, unstructured interviews were carried out with a number of individual alcoholics and non-alcoholics, who were all questioned about the relationship between their jobs and their drinking. Some of these conversations were tape recorded, and taped material was collected from subjects who between them had experience of the following occupations: musician, teacher, executive, journalist, writer, television producer, doctor, skilled building worker, power station operator, labourer, engineer, merchant seaman. In addition, the investigator accompanied a salesman when entertaining customers, and thus gained first-hand experience of the meaning of drink in that situation.

From analysis of this pre-pilot material it was possible further to identify the processes which might (across occupations) be seen as common and fundamental to genesis of drinking pressures. In the pilot stage a questionnaire was developed by repeated administration to individuals or small groups, and subsequent discussion with those who completed the questionnaires, and a key section was built to deal with these identified drink-related processes. The six questions finally chosen as comprising the 'occupational sub-factors' enquiry were:

1   Have you been able to get drinks cheaply or free on most weeks at work for a period of one year or more? (Do not include meths.)

2   Have you been involved in the making, distribution or sale of alcohol for a period of one year or more?

3   Have you had an entertaining allowance or expense account at work for a period of one year or more?

4   Have you travelled away from home most weeks, or lived abroad because of work for a period of one year or more?

5   Have you used drink to aid business contacts on most weeks for a period of one year or more?

6   Have you worked where most employers drank at work for a period of one year or more?

Other key sections of questionnaire-building related to drinking history, drinking attitudes and occupational history.

11 Appraisal

The studies reported in this section are all to a degree essays in the same research style. The style at first glance might perhaps be identified as that of the relatively atheoretical and descriptive questionnaire-based study of the special (and to an extent 'atypical') population. Such an approach is perhaps today not an altogether popular one, and the professional social scientist will rather easily insert the word 'merely' before the word 'descriptive'.

Criticisms of this type of research strategy go under a number of headings. There is firstly the point that seemingly atheoretical research is never truly designed without covert theoretical assumptions; some hidden preconceptions are always there, and these are vital determinants of the researcher's choice of what he puts into or leaves out of his questionnaire. The fault is not that the design is atheoretical, but that the theory is a hazy and only half-spelled out one. In consequence questions vital to the investigator's concern may go unasked, while at the same time the questionnaire may be overloaded with much which in no way serves the hidden purpose. Such criticisms could perhaps be levelled for instance at the study of London's Skid Row. What is the purpose of asking about religious affiliation? Why wasn't enquiry into help-seeking behaviour much more detailed?

A second criticism would be that the use of a semi-structured or structured questionnaire is inappropriate at this stage of investigation. If we admit that all these efforts to look at special groups are basically only of a very exploratory nature, why accept the constraining formality of the questionnaire? There are certainly other investigative techniques available, and the sociologist who is interested in the difficult and demanding techniques of participant observation, might well suggest that the trained and sensitive observer who lived for a few months in a reception centre might come back with more insights than did the bevy of interlopers who (questionnaires in hand) briefly raided the place on one particular evening.

Objection might then also be made to the uncertainty which inevitably attaches to interpretation of any results which came from the study of a sample of alcoholics as special as those who are to be found in a particular recidivist prison, as egregious as AA attenders or members of the Renaissance Group. What price extrapolation?

These and other criticisms deserve careful attention. There are, on the other hand, some few points which should be made in support of the other side in this debate. Here it might be interesting to start with what might be considered

77

a 'political' rather than a research perspective: the focused descriptive study on an atypical group may in fact be focusing on a population which is of very immediate societal concern, a population about which even the rudiments of descriptive information may be astonishingly lacking and societal misconceptions rife, and the research report may have immediate relevance to society's decision making. The work on Skid Row and on the drunkenness offender which is reported here had direct effect on the setting up of community facilities, and probably to a modest extent (along with much work from research centres other than the Addiction Research Unit) bore on the recommendations which the Home Office Working Party on the Habitual Drunkenness Offender felt able to make.

The most important point which has to be made is probably that the polarity is a false one: this type of small focused project properly conducted is not the enemy of theoretically based research. The criticisms are properly not those of the research style itself but of that style if it is poorly executed. The whole concept of 'this' style of research becomes hazy, its boundaries unclear, once the critics' point is accepted that all work is to a degree theoretically based. The attack is in truth not on any particular research style, but simply on any research which is carelessly conceived and which has insufficient definition of assumption or of purpose.

In these days of the large population survey, the seductions of the computer, the big research team, the expensive budget and often the absurdly prolonged gap between the launching of the project and the report reaching the relevant desks, there is a case for further definition of the ground rules for the small-scale study of special populations, but it would be a pity if such studies were swept out of fashion.

Part III   Hospital treatment studies

12   Hypnosis in treatment of alcohol addiction: Controlled trial, with analysis of factors affecting outcome *

GRIFFITH EDWARDS

Summary

Forty alcoholics were randomised between a conventional treatment régime and conventional treatment plus hypnosis. At 12 months from hospital discharge there was no difference in outcome between the two groups. A social stability score was highly prognostic of outcome and two personality measures less so.

Results are compared in two groups of patients – one which received the usual in-patient treatment régime employed at the Maudsley Hospital, and another which in addition was given hypnotic treatment. The hypothesis to be tested was that hypnosis is a valuable adjunct to conventional treatment.

Method

Randomisation. When a pair of patients had been found who, on clinical assessment were thought to have roughly the same prognosis, a coin was spun and one was allocated to the non-hypnotic group while the other was allocated to the hypnotic group. This process was repeated until there were 20 matched pairs.

Treatment: non-hypnotic group. The essential background to all treatment was admission to a general psychiatric ward. More specific measures included individual psychotherapy largely directed at the patient's immediate problems, disulfiram, Alcoholics Anonymous and social rehabilitation.

Treatment: hypnotic group. These patients received the same treatment as

---

* Synopsis of a paper of the same title, originally appearing in the *Quarterly Journal of Studies on Alcohol,* vol. 15, 1966, pp. 147–9.

those in the control group but in addition hypnosis was employed. Carefully defined post-hypnotic suggestions were given of:

(a) a distaste for alcohol; a wish to maintain abstinence, a sense of accomplishment and increased well-being stemming from sobriety;
(b) a determination to continue taking disulfiram with unfailing regularity; and
(c) an interest in AA which would result in continued attendance at meetings.

Therapeutic post-hypnotic suggestion was given on six consecutive days and was then re-inforced at weekly intervals during the patient's stay in hospital.
Follow-up. Patients were asked to attend a clinic at not less than monthly intervals for the first six months, and thereafter to attend not less often than every two months, until a year after discharge from the ward. With all patients emphasis was put on the necessity for continued abstinence, and on the need to go on attending AA and taking disulfiram. In the hypnotic group, therapeutic post-hypnotic suggestion was repeated at monthly intervals for the first six months.
Ratings. Social stability (SS) for the period immediately preceding admission to hospital was scored on the 4-point scale described by Straus and Bacon (1951); neuroticism (N) and extraversion (E) were measured on the MPI (Eysenck 1959). Treatment outcome was rated at monthly intervals during the 12 months after discharge. Each month either an A (2-point), a B (1-point) or a C (zero) rating was given. Details of this system of assessment were as follows:

A Completely sober for the month under consideration, or occasional drinking (less than seven days out of the whole month), without there being interference with social functioning.
B Drinking more than occasionally (more than seven days out of the month) or occasional drinking causing mild social incapacity (e.g., patient missing a few days' work).
C Drinking heavily, with drinking causing considerable social incapacity, e.g., prolonged unemployment, hospitalisation or imprisonment.

Results

Monthly assessment. There was no significant difference between the two groups. In both groups the first six months saw the majority of relapses with few further relapses in the second six months.
Overall assessments for year. By summing monthly scores for 12 months, an

overall score was calculated for each patient; the maximum score for any patient was thus 12 × A, i.e., 12 × 2 points. The categories for the year's outcome were defined as: I = Good = Score 17–24; II = Fair = Score 9–16; III = Poor = Score 0–8. In the hypnotic and control groups identical results were obtained: I – 11 patients; II – 2 patients; and III – 7 patients.

Analysis of factors affecting outcome in combined hypnotic and control groups. For purpose of further statistical analysis, the assumption was made that hypnotic and control group patients could be treated as one population. Neuroticism has a significant negative correlation with outcome ($p < .05$); extraversion has a significant positive correlation with outcome ($p < .05$); and social stability has a highly significant positive correlation with outcome ($p < .001$). Extraversion and neuroticism were not completely independent but showed a negative correlation; social stability was negatively correlated with neuroticism and positively correlated with extraversion.

The contributions of extraversion, neuroticism and social stability to the total variance of outcome score were then examined in an analysis of variance. The contribution of extraversion to the total variance was very slight; a regression equation was therefore calculated using neuroticism and social stability only. This equation is:

$$SS \times 4.157 - N \times 0.021 + 5.376 = OS.$$

It can be seen that in this equation a change of 50 units in the neuroticism score is needed to produce a change of one unit in outcome score.

Regularity of AA attendance. There was no evidence to suggest that the two groups differed in any way in AA attendance.

Regularity in taking disulfiram. There was again no difference between the two groups.

Discussion

Value of hypnosis in the treatment of alcoholism. The trial demonstrates that when hypnotic treatment is added to conventional treatment no advantage is conferred – a conclusion which contrasts with claims which have been made for the efficacy of hypnotic treatment of alcoholism when those claims have rested on clinical impression rather than on controlled experimentation.

What is social stability? Social stability, as measured on the Straus-Bacon scale, correlates highly with outcome. Implications of this finding depend on whether social stability is simply a reflection of personality or of drinking history, or whether alternatively it is to be considered a variable to an important extent independent of these other factors. The only satisfactory explanation of its basis seems to be that very many different factors are contributory. These factors are personality-determined as well as environment-determined, and drink-determined as well as being unrelated to the drinking. To analyse separately all these factors would present a considerable task, and it is fortunate therefore that their end product, the social stability score which is easily obtained, is so good a guide to outcome. That initial social stability is correlated with outcome may bear on the emphasis which is to be given to the patient's immediate social problems in the total treatment. Such a correlation is of course no proof that treatment with greater emphasis on improving social stability would result in improved outcome, but the finding does suggest leads which should be pursued in clinical investigation. Comparison of groups of patients with whom emphasis was placed on environmental manipulation or psychotherapy alternatively, would be of great interest.

The advantage of using a precise mathematical method in analysing results is apparent, for although the paper by Davies et al., (1956) demonstrated that both social stability and personality were of importance in impact on prognosis, the method they used could not give any measure of the relative importance of these different factors. Application of statistical methods and further planned investigation can be expected to give information which should help greatly in planning the optimum treatment for the individual patient.

13 A controlled trial of inpatient and outpatient treatment of alcohol dependency*

GRIFFITH EDWARDS and SALLY GUTHRIE

Summary

Forty alcohol-dependent men who had no other severe physical or mental illness and who agreed to accept either treatment were randomised to inpatient or outpatient therapy. The average stay in hospital was 8.9 weeks for inpatients, while outpatients on average spent 7.7 weeks in 'intensive treatment'. A correlation analysis showed a relation between demographic and personality factors, drinking chronology, and 'complications of drinking' but did not reveal any significant prognostic factors. All patients were followed up to one year with monthly assessment of progress made on a two-point scale by independent raters. There was no significant difference between groups. The bearing of these results on the planning of future treatment is discussed and it is suggested that emphasis should be on development of the comprehensive treatment service, which would integrate inpatient and outpatient services and also provide hostel care. The specialised inpatient unit is probably of value, but criteria for admission need to be much more strictly defined.

Introduction

The specialised treatment of alcohol dependence (addiction) in the UK usually starts with the patient spending some weeks in hospital. Table 13.1 shows the duration of admission reported in six series of alcoholics treated in Britain.

The Ministry of Health (1962) proposed that the specialised inpatient unit should be the mainstay of alcoholism treatment services, and 13 of these units are now in existence. Probably, all would agree that subsequent aftercare is vital. The World Health Organisation's (1951) emphasis on the importance of outpatient clinics has, in England and Wales, received relatively little attention.

Is there indeed any firm evidence that this initial period in hospital really

---

* A slightly shortened version of a paper of the same title, originally appearing in the *Lancet,* vol. 1, 1967, pp. 555–9.

Table 13.1
Duration of inpatient stay in six British series

Reference	Place of treatment	Duration of inpatient stay
Glatt (1955)	Warlingham Park: specialised alcoholism unit	At least 2 months: 'on the whole about 3 months is the optimum period'.
Davies et al. (1956)	Maudsley: general psychiatric ward	2–3 months but up to 10 months in one case
Vallance (1965)	Southern General, Glasgow: general psychiatric unit	2–3 weeks average
Edwards (1966)	Maudsley: general psychiatric ward	about 8 weeks average
Rathod et al. (1966)	Warlingham Park: specialised alcoholism unit	10–14 weeks
Walton et al. (1966)	Royal Edinburgh: specialised alcoholism unit	3–4 weeks

affects the long term outcome? Or would most alcoholics do equally well if they were from the start offered no more than energetic outpatient treatment? This question is of importance to the National Health Service – the World Health Organisation's (1951) provisional estimate in 1948 was of very roughly 350,000 alcoholics, about 75,000 of these being 'chronic alcoholics', in England and Wales. A Ministry which is responsible for organising treatment services on this scale will face a heavy bill if therapy is to mean eight to 12 weeks in the wards.

Objective evaluation of different regimens with alcoholics randomly allocated to treatment groups has very seldom been undertaken. Wallerstein (1957) compared four inpatient treatment methods and Bruun (1963) and Bahn et al. (1963) assessed different types of alcoholism clinic. Chafetz (1961) randomised patients between two types of intake procedure. However, the efficacy of outpatient as opposed to inpatient care remains as open a question in alcoholism as in the treatment of most other psychiatric conditions. The criteria on which a neurotic receives inpatient, day hospital, or outpatient care might, for instance, be stated with some agreement by experienced psychiatrists, but objective appraisal of the correctness of these criteria on which such important (and expensive) decisions are made is very largely lacking. In planning psychiatric services, studies of alcoholism, a disease in which outcome is relatively easily measured, can perhaps in some ways provide a model.

Methods

Admission to the trial and randomisation

All patients were men who gave a history of drinking being 'out of control', and had symptoms of chemical dependence on alcohol: the picture conformed to that of the 'gamma alcoholism' syndrome of Jellinek's (1960) typology and the illness was in all cases of such severity as would normally have been considered as an indication for a full course of inpatient treatment. Because the trial was concerned with dependence rather than with the acute physical or mental complications of alcoholism, patients who had, for instance, delirium tremens, might enter the series after a few days in an observation ward. Presence of other severe physical or mental disease was a disqualification, and vagrant alcoholics of Skid Row type were excluded.

When each of the above criteria had been met, each patient was asked whether he would accept with equal willingness either treatment (inpatient or outpatient) which might be offered, and only then was randomisation made. Two patients who were offered treatment refused to accept this imposed condition, both of them objecting to the possibility of hospitalisation; it seems likely that this clause did not therefore materially influence the definition of the sample or bias it towards specially co-operative cases. There were 20 patients in each treatment group.

Treatment

Treatment was to some extent varied according to the individual patient's needs rather than being dictated by an unrealistically rigid treatment schedule, but this variation was kept within as narrow limits as were consistent with competent therapy.

Inpatient group. Patients were admitted to a 30-bed general psychiatric ward in which there were four or five alcoholics. The treatment regimen was eclectic. Withdrawal symptoms were, when necessary, covered with a tranquilliser, but patients were not kept on long term treatment with these drugs. Central importance was given to the doctor forming a good relationship with the patient. Discussion included repeated exploration of the reasons for drinking and of possible alternative methods of dealing with anxiety or anger, and immediate reality problems received attention. Dogmatic emphasis was put on alcohol dependence being a disease completely precluding return to social drinking. Patients were encouraged to attend meetings of Alcoholics Anonymous and an AA sponsor accompanied patients to meetings of local groups. Every patient received citrated calcium carbimide ('Abstem') 100 mg. per day, and a test reaction was carried out. A social worker helped with employment and other social problems, and when necessary undertook family case-work. The length of stay in hospital was intended to be approximately eight weeks. After discharge patients were seen at least once each month.

Outpatient group. Outpatients received a very similar treatment, except that stress was placed on the need to regard alcoholism as an illness which could be met without retreat to hospital and without avoidance of any social responsibilities. Patients were encouraged to return to work as soon as possible. Withdrawal symptoms were to be dealt with at home with the help of general practitioner, family, and AA sponsor. Psychotherapy and social work were part of the regimen as with the inpatients, and if a patient failed to keep an appointment, a social worker would make immediate contact with the home. An abstem test reaction was carried out, with overnight admission to hospital for this purpose. The initial 'intensive treatment' period was planned as being of about eight weeks, and during this time patients were seen not less than once fortnightly; thereafter, as with the discharged inpatients, outpatients were seen not less than once monthly.

Assessment

Inpatients were assessed at monthly intervals after discharge while outpatients were assessed at monthly intervals from the end of the period of intensive care. In nearly all instances the patients' statements were verified by independent evidence from wife or employer. Using all the available evidence, each of us made a separate rating for each month's outcome:

2 points: completely sober for the month under consideration or occasional drinking (less than seven days in the month) without interference with social function.

1 point: drinking more than occasionally (more than seven days in the month) or drinking occasionally causing mild social incapacity (e.g., patient missing a

86

few days' work).

0 points: heavy drinking causing considerable social incapacity (e.g., prolonged unemployment, hospitalisation or imprisonment).

A patient could thus score 0–24 points on the year's follow-up.

Results

Characteristics of patients and matching of groups

Marital status. Twelve of the inpatients and 16 of the outpatients were married and living with wife, two in either group were single, and six inpatients and two outpatients were separated or divorced.

Social class was categorised in terms of the Registrar General's Classification of Occupations (General Register Office, 1960) and distribution is shown in Table 13.2. The difference in class distribution is not significant.

Table 13.2
Social class

Class	Inpatients	Outpatients
I (professional)	0	1
II	5	5
III	10	8
IV	1	3
V (unskilled labour)	4	3

Social stability was rated on a 4-point scale derived from Straus and Bacon (1951), to give a measure of 'social rootedness'. The mean score of the inpatient group was 2.35 and for the outpatient group 2.95: the difference is not significant.

Drinking history. Table 13.3 is based on information given by patients in answer to specific enquiry on initial assessment. The two groups do not differ significantly.

Personality and intelligence. Each patient completed the Maudsley Personality Inventory (Eysenck 1959): mean N (neuroticism) score was 34 for inpatients and 36 for outpatients, and mean E (extraversion) 24 for either group. The IQ score on the Mill Hill vocabulary test was 106 for inpatients and 108 for outpatient group, and on Raven's progressive matrices 111 for

87

Table 13.3
Chronology of drinking history

Event	Mean age (years)	
	Inpatient	Outpatient
First took a drink	15	16
First got drunk	18	21
First drinking most days	24	29
Drinking first caused damage	31	33
Patient first saw drinking as problem	35	39
This admission	42	44

either group.

Daily alcohol consumption. Average stated daily alcohol consumption was (very approximately) equivalent to 500 ml. per day and 480 ml. per day absolute alcohol for inpatients and outpatients, respectively; these levels do not differ significantly.

Correlation analysis

A 30 × 30 item-correlation matrix was prepared to examine relations between demographic and personality factors, drinking chronology, 'complications of drinking', and outcome. An abstract from this matrix, giving a 15 × 6 matrix, is given in Table 13.4. The main findings were that none of the items analysed had a significant bearing on outcome but that personality, intelligence, and social factors were significantly related to occurrence of 'complications' and to drinking history.

A higher N score, for instance, did not militate against success in treatment, but meant that a patient was likely to have come to treatment earlier, to have developed a drinking problem earlier in life, to have a higher probability of experiencing amnesias, of being charged for drunkenness, and of having pawned.

Length of treatment

The average stay in hospital was 8.9 weeks for inpatients while outpatients on average spent 7.7 weeks in 'intensive treatment' with 7.5 clinic visits during that period.

Table 13.4
Extract from correlation matrix

Item	Significance of correlation with item					
	1	2	3	4	5	6
1 N						
2 IQ verbal						
3 Married						
4 Age	− −	+ + +				
5 Age first problem	−	+		+ + +		
6 Social stability			+	+	+	
7 Higher class		+ + +	+	+ +		
8 Daily alcohol	−			−	−	
9 Early-morning drink						−
10 Amnesias	+					−
11 Suicidal attempt						−
12 Drunk charge	+ + +	−		−		
13 Pawning	+ +		−			
14 Previous treatment			−			
15 Outcome score						

Significant positive correlation marked:+ (P<0.05), + + (P<0.01), and + + + (P<0.001), with similar notation for significance of negative correlations.

Outcome

Outcome ratings. Scoring by the two raters was identical in all but 13 of the 480 monthly ratings: the categories were meaningful and easy to apply. Where there was a discrepancy the mean of two ratings was taken.

Monthly group outcomes (maximum 20×2 points) were calculated for each group, and the results are given in Table 13.5: the two groups followed rather parallel courses, with the outpatient group seeming to have some slight advantage. Analysis of variance (Table 13.6) shows, however, that neither between-treatment variance nor the interaction between months and treatment is significant.

Table 13.7 shows the outcome at the end of one year, broken down in detail, with the number of patients in each group who scored 0, 1, or 2 points in the twelfth month. The comparison here again confirms that there is no significant difference in outcome between the two groups.

Table 13.5
Group scores for each of 12 follow-up months

Group	Group score at month											
	1	2	3	4	5	6	7	8	9	10	11	12
Inpatient	32	28	29	27	24	21	21	21	23	22.5	21.5	23
Outpatient	32	28	29.5	27.5	28.5	25	28	30.5	29.5	28.5	30	25.5

Table 13.6
Outcome scores: analysis of variance

Variance	Degrees of freedom	Sum of squares	Mean sum of squares	Variance ratio	Signifi-cance (P)
Between Patients:	39	202.93	–	–	–
Between treatment	1	5.10	5.10	0.98	–
Residual	38	197.83	5.21	–	–
Within Patients:	440	148.44	–	–	–
Between months	11	6.83	0.621	1.85	0.05
Months × treatment	11	1.76	0.160	0.48	–
Residual	418	139.85	0.335	–	–
Total	479	–	–	–	–

Table 13.7
Outcome at 1 year: number of patients in each category

Group	No. with score		
	0	1	2
Inpatient	7	3	10
Outpatient	4	6	10

Use of hostels

Six former inpatients and four of the outpatients were resident in special alcoholism rehabilitation hostels during some part of the follow-up year. The average period of residence was 19 and 12 weeks, respectively.

Hospital admission during the follow-up year

Four of the inpatient group and three of the outpatients were, during the follow-up year, admitted to observation wards or to general hospitals for a few days, while two and one of inpatient and outpatient groups, respectively, were admitted to mental hospital for some weeks of treatment: the patient from the outpatient group admitted to a mental hospital continued to score 0 after discharge. There was thus no evidence that during the follow-up year greater use had to be made of hospital admission by patients in the outpatient group than by those who had received an initial period of inpatient treatment.

Discussion

Comparability of groups

In no respect did the characteristics of the two groups differ significantly. The slight excess of divorced or separated men in the inpatient group, which is reflected in a correspondingly slightly lower social stability score, is, on the evidence of the correlation analysis, unlikely to have had any adverse bias on the inpatient group outcome.

Treatment outcome

Interpretation of the results should not go beyond the statements that a *certain type* of outpatient treatment has been shown, on average, to give as good results as a *certain type* of inpatient treatment: there remain inevitable difficulties in deciding how far extrapolation is justified from treatment results obtained with the particular regimens used at one hospital to wide conclusions on the intrinsic merits of inpatient as compared to outpatient treatment in general. Champions of inpatient treatment might argue that the answer would have been different if the inpatient regimen had been centred on intensive group psychotherapy but, despite the current popularity of group methods, there is little evidence that individual treatment gives inferior results: the outcomes reported in two important English series employing respectively group (Glatt, 1961b) and individual (Davies et al., 1956) regimens were similar, and the patient-populations probably roughly comparable.

One advantage of outpatient treatment is that the wife can take credit for success rather than her having the wounding experience of her husband being abruptly taken into hospital, later to return as the hospital's success and as a strange sober man suddenly demanding a new and dominant role within the home. In other ways, too, outpatient treatment seems to mobilise help – the general practitioner can be the key figure in successful outpatient care, and a patient is quick to appreciate the help which AA can give when a sponsor visits him at home and sits with him through his withdrawal symptoms.

To interpret this trial as showing that inpatient treatment of alcohol addiction is never indicated would certainly be too sweeping: the similarity of inpatient and outpatient results could mask particular subgroups of patients for whom one or other treatment is more suitable, and there is a need for clinical trials which aim at investigating the *specific* indications for one or other type of treatment. There are, in all probability, patients who will benefit from two to three months respite in hospital with forced removal from drinking, and who would not recover if left in the disorganised social setting with which they can no longer cope; and in future analyses the effects of hospital admission *per se* and of psychotherapy should be separately assessed. We do not believe that our findings undermine the position of the specialist inpatient units, but rather suggest that they point to the need for the alcoholism treatment systems to be expanded so that these units form part of a properly comprehensive service.

A comprehensive alcoholism treatment service

The essence of treatment of alcoholism is often the long-term support of someone who is going to be repeatedly in trouble. At present, the state of affairs facing a GP who wants help with an alcoholic is often deplorable and the backing which a specialised service can provide for him ought to be a measure of its efficiency. Waiting lists are frequently long, and when the patient is eventually seen, the expert opinion may be that he is unsuitable for the alcoholism unit, and the case is back on the GP's hands. The GP may then get his patient into the local area hospital but the Ministry's plea to regional boards that they should establish specialised units is in some ways an admission that NHS mental hospitals are not always able to give the type of help required. A GP may find it hard to locate a hospital bed for 'drying out' for a patient who has been doing well but requires brief admission to cut short a drinking bout.

A treatment service should integrate the whole range of help which is required if every type of alcoholic is to receive treatment – from the initial emergency aid to long-term rehabilitation.

The pivot of the service should be an *alcoholism emergency clinic* which would see new cases at any time (night or day, weekday or weekend), referred from any source or self-referred, and would also see at short notice any patient who had relapsed. This clinic would then refer the case to one of the other six integrated services.

Alcoholism treatment clinic. Patients would be referred to this clinic direct from their GP if not urgent, or otherwise via the alcoholism emergency clinic. The clinic would give intensive or supportive treatment and would accept responsibility for follow-up care of discharged patients.

Emergency beds. A small number of emergency beds would be available for 'drying out'; these could be used either for new cases seen in the emergency clinic, or for old patients who had relapsed.

Inpatient treatment beds. Alcoholics are perhaps best treated in a special ward, which can be organised along the lines of a therapeutic community, but it must be noted that in some hospitals this has not been found necessary.

Hostels. Hostel care may be needed for any patient who is without good social support: patients can be admitted direct to a hostel while undergoing outpatient treatment or could be admitted after discharge from the wards. It is likely that the treatment service would need to establish several hostels for patients with different needs – one hostel, for instance, might offer long-term (or life-time) support for the Skid Row alcoholic (Myerson, 1956) while another hostel might evolve a more dynamic group (Edwards et al., 1966a).

Referral out. Patients would have to be referred out from the alcoholism treatment service for certain specialised purposes, e.g., intensive individual psychotherapy, long-term care of the alcoholic dement.

Community liaison. The treatment service should have close liaison with all community resources, both statutory and voluntary. Evans et al. (1966) have shown how valuable the link can be with local authority resources. Co-operation with Alcoholics Anonymous is essential. An active community council on alcoholism which would increase public awareness of this disease should be fostered, and an information centre of the kind sponsored by the National Council on Alcoholism (Perceval, 1966) can do much to stimulate community interest.

A treatment service providing for the needs of an urban area should have its alcoholism emergency clinic, its drying-out beds, its alcoholism treatment clinic, and its hostels as centrally situated as would be expected of general surgical or general medical services. Central siting of the inpatient treatment beds is not so vital.

From the patient's point of view the obvious advantage of a properly integrated alcoholism treatment service is that he will be in contact with the same person throughout treatment and rehabilitation. Organising such a comprehensive service would be a considerable task, and the consultant in charge of the service would probably be engaged in this work for the major part of his time. There is, however, a case to be made for ensuring that alcoholism treatment does not become a closed cult. One of the tasks of the specialist is to show all his colleagues that anyone who acquires the necessary skills has a part to play in the treatment of this disease.

Cost is important: a co-ordinated service as envisaged here would be largely a matter of more effective, rather than more expensive, redeployment of resources which are today being used wastefully. Some additional expense would be incurred by the engagement of extra psychiatric social workers and provision for consultant sessions, but cost to the country might well be offset if a disease which debits industry by millions of pounds a year (National Council on Alcoholism, 1965) were more successfully treated.

14 Metronidazole in the treatment of alcohol addiction: a controlled trial*

M. G. GELDER and GRIFFITH EDWARDS

Summary

The supposed adverse properties of metronidazole were examined in a trial which used ten patients as their own controls. Semantic differential ratings of attitudes toward drink were employed. The drug produced no disulfiram-like effect, but appeared to interfere with the taste of alcohol.

Procedure

A double-blind controlled trial investigated the possible disulfiram-like effects of metronidazole, and its ability to reduce craving.

Ten patients took part; all were gamma alcoholics in Jellinek's (1960) classification. Each patient took metronidazole 400 mg. four times a day for ten days, and an identical placebo for ten days, the order of administration being randomised. An alcohol test was carried out at the end of each ten day period, and baseline measurements were obtained before any drugs were taken. The alcohol test followed the usual lines of an alcohol antabuse test. In addition, both patient and psychiatrist filled in a questionnaire about the signs and symptoms which might be expected to follow if metronidazole produced an alcohol-antabuse-like reaction.

Craving was assessed indirectly, using a form of semantic differential test (Marks, 1965); ratings on seven point scales were combined to give five 'factor' scores: evaluation, potency, flavour, danger and anxiety.

Results

Disulfiram-like effects

After the test dose of alcohol, the slight fall of standing and lying blood pressure and pulse rate was not significantly different after placebo and metronidazole. There was also no significant difference in the number of

---

* Synopsis of a paper of the same title which originally appeared in the *British Journal of Psychiatry,* vol. 114, 1968, pp. 473–5.

Table 14.1
Ratings of 'The drink you are offering me now'; 'the drink I have just taken';
and 'a further drink if offered'

				'Factor' Scores		
		Eval.	Potency	Flavour	Danger	Anxiety
I	A drink if offered me now					
	(Day 1)	3.0	4.6	3.8	5.6	3.3
II	Drink you are offering me now					
	(a) after placebo	3.5	4.4	3.8	4.4	3.5
	(b) after metronidazole	3.5	4.4	4.0	3.7	2.1*
III	Drink I have just taken					
	(a) after placebo	2.0	3.2	2.5	3.6‡	2.5
	(b) after metronidazole	2.4	3.6	2.9	3.7‡	2.7
IV	A further drink if offered					
	(a) after placebo	2.2	3.8	2.3*	3.4†	2.4
	(b) after metronidazole	2.4	3.8	2.9	4.2*	2.7

* Differs beyond 0.5 per cent level from corresponding factor of I.
† Differs beyond 0.1 per cent level from corresponding factor of I.
‡ Differs beyond 0.01 per cent level from corresponding factor of I.

positive items on the check lists after metronidazole and placebo.

Semantic differential (Table 14.1)

The two control concepts did not change significantly during the 21 days of the trial. The patients rated a 'drink if offered me now' on the first day: it was expected to be mildly pleasant, neutral as regards potency and flavour, moderately dangerous and slightly calming. This as a base-line against which other ratings were compared.

'The drink you are offering me now' was related immediately before the test dose of alcohol. After metronidazole it was rated more calming than the baseline expectation ($p < .05$), no other comparisons were significant, and no significant changes occurred after placebo.

'The drink I have just taken' rated immediately after the test drink, was rated significantly less dangerous than the baseline expectation, after both

metronidazole and placebo. The ratings of evaluation, potency and flavour all became more favourable after taking the drink, both in metronidazole and placebo groups.

'A further drink if offered me now' was rated immediately after the test drink and is an indirect measure of craving for another drink. Again it was significantly less dangerous than the baseline expectation after both drug and placebo, although the change was less after metronidazole. After placebo it was rated significantly better in flavour, but this change was less after metronidazole and did not reach significance.

Patients' spontaneous comments were recorded. They were strikingly similar after drug and placebo and patients were unanimous in regarding the effect of the metronidazole–alcohol reaction as mild and extremely unlikely to deter them from drinking.

Discussion

It is of interest that complaints that drinks tasted bitter after metronidazole were recorded by Semer et al. (1966), and bad taste in the mouth was reported by Bonfiglio and Donadio (1966) and Blom (1967). These other authors regarded these as 'side-effects'. We suggest they may be one of the main effects of the drug in relation to alcoholism. The recent finding that taste is an important determinant of alcohol choice in rats (Lester, 1966) may be relevant here, and comparable systematic findings should perhaps be carried out in man.

Reports that some patients have been able to drink socially after metronidazole may be further evidence that some alcohol addicts can return to normal drinking (Davies, 1962; Kendell, 1965), rather than of any specific effect of the drug.

The drug deserves further study, as the ways in which it leads to sedation and influences flavour are not understood. We do not, however, consider that the present evidence justifies its use in the treatment of alcoholism.

15 Life events and alcoholic relapse*

BRIAN D. HORE

Summary

A six month prospective study of a group of alcoholics is described who were closely followed up with a view to determining the relationship between life events and relapse into drinking. It seems likely that for some patients such environmental factors were of considerable importance in precipitating relapse, while other patients who encountered much the same sort of stress did not drink.

Introduction

The study of the relationships between life events and the onset or exacerbation of psychiatric illness has gained increasing importance in recent years (Adamson and Schmale, 1965; Brown and Birley, 1968; Cassidy et al., 1957; Forrest et al., 1965; Hudgens et al., 1967). Such studies have inherent problems. These include retrospective falsification, the question of which events to include and the difficulty of distinguishing between precipitating events and events induced by illness itself. It is perhaps not surprising that results have been conflicting and opinions range from those who see a causal relationship to those who see only a relationship explicable by chance. A comparative view of the literature is hindered by the fact that many authors fail to list the types of events included, although there are exceptions (Adamson and Schmale, 1965). Two studies deserve further mention as they have attempted to overcome some of the problems above. Rahe (1968) has attempted a prospective study using naval personnel and found preceding life events could have a predictive value in assessing the likelihood of future illnesses, whilst Brown and Birley (1968) in their study of schizophrenic patients have introduced the concept of independent life events as a category of events that could not have been brought about by the patient himself; they classify their events into two, independent events, and all others are called possibly independent. Amongst those who have claimed a causal link between

---

* This paper originally appeared in the *British Journal of Addiction*, vol. 66, 1971, pp. 83–8.

life events and onset of exacerbation of psychiatric illness there has been agreement that events of a personal intimate kind, such as difficulties in interpersonal relationships, are of the greatest importance.

Although a wide range of psychiatric disorder has been studied in this way there appears to have been no systematic study of the relationship between events in the lives of alcoholics and episodes of relapse into drinking, although relapse is very frequent and at least in some alcoholics a relationship would appear possible. The present investigation is a prospective study of a group of 28 alcoholics followed for periods of up to six months in which regular assessment was made of life events and episodes of relapse. Events were assessed by two methods, clinical interview and the use of the Brown and Birley structured events questionnaire (Brown and Birley, 1968); in this way it was hoped to avoid the problem of either only including very 'hard' data or of including all events, together with those of a symbolic nature (Adamson and Schmale, 1965).

Method

The procedure is explained in detail elsewhere (Hore, 1971). Here only the essentials will be given. The patients were either alcoholic outpatients currently attending the Maudsley Hospital (25) or inpatients in a psychiatric unit in a general hospital (three). The latter were followed from their discharge from hospital. All patients satisfied the WHO 1952 definition of alcoholism. Patients were seen at weekly intervals for periods up to six months. Careful recording was made from the patients and then relatives of any period of relapse; this was defined as either any drinking (the majority) or as any increase in drinking outside their social norm (two patients). At the weekly visit each patient was asked as part of the clinical interview to relate any events in his life; and at monthly intervals he was given the Brown and Birley questionnaire; this is a systematic enquiry into the presence or absence of events in the patient's life which does not ask reactions to events, but rather lists the presence or absence of events themselves. The events included are those the authors feel on commonsense grounds would be likely to produce emotional disturbance in most people and, as outlined above, are divided into independent and possibly dependent. Where possible, relatives were seen at weekly and monthly intervals and asked similar questions regarding life events.

Results

As stated above 28 patients began the study but six broke off within one month, and data was therefore only recorded on 22. Four patients did not relapse, and in a further four there was considerable doubt as to accurate dating of relapse and life events. In the remaining 14 patients, in whom it was felt data was recorded accurately, there were 41 episodes of relapse and 52 events. The type of events occurring and their temporal relationship to relapse is shown in Table 15.1.

Table 15.1

Summary of events and their temporal relationships to relapse in 14 patients

Patient number	Description of events	Date of events from onset of study in weeks	Date of relapse from onset of study in weeks	Follow-up no. of weeks
1	(1) Quarrel with homosexual partner	2nd	(1) 3rd	
	(2) Homosexual partner went on holiday	6th	(2) 7th	
	(3) Homosexual partner went on holiday	14th	(3) 14th	
	(4) Quarrel with homosexual partner	15th	(4) 15th	26
	(5) Homosexual partner threatened to get married	16th	(5) 17th	
	(6) Quarrel with homosexual partner	19th	(6) 19th	
	(7) Quarrel with homosexual partner	20th	(7) 20th	
4	(1) Restarted work after 5 weeks off	2nd	(1) 22nd	
	(2) Changed job	8th		
	(3) Application for council housing refused	10th		24
	(4) Temporary promotion to chargehand	16th		
	(5) Birth of first grandchild	18th		
5	(1) Husband aged 30 admitted to hospital (diagnosis pneumonia)		(1) 3rd	
			(2) 6th	
		24th	(3) 16th	26
			(4) 19th	
			(5) 21st	
			(6) 25th	
6	(1) Met new girl friend	13th	(1) 14th	
	(2) Not allowed at the last minute to take children on holiday (patient's divorced wife has custody of the children)	16th	(2) 17th	23
			(3) 23rd	
7	(1) Discharge from general hospital	4th	(1) 6th	
	(2) Moved lodgings	9th	(2) 14th	
	(3) Started new job after 3 months' unemployment	19th	(3) 19th	31
	(4) Broke ankle at work	19th	(4) 26th	
			(5) 31st	

8			20th	26
10	(1) Failed driving test and lost potential job	1st		
	(2) Severe quarrels with wife	7th/8th	(1) 8th	
	(3) Threw up job	8th		
	(4) Restarted work	15th		
	(5) Visited parents in Birmingham – family row	20th		30
	(6) Told job redundancy very likely	21st	(2) 21st	
	(7) Father and father's mistress paid a surprise visit	26th	(3) 26th	
			(4) 30th	
11	(1) Request for job transfer granted	8th	(1) 3rd	26
	(2) Restarted work after 3 months' off	18th		
12	(1) Restarted work after 8 weeks	6th		
	(2) Changed job	8th		23
	(3) Restarted work after hospital inpatient treatment (2 weeks)	20th	(1) 14th	
	(4) Move to alcoholic hostel	23rd	(2) 18th	
13	(1) Sister-in-law (household member) had first baby	12th	(1) 7th	13
	(2) Returned to work after 6 weeks off	13th		
15	(1) First grandchild born	4th		
	(2) Major row with foreman	8th		
	(3) Son left home for first time	12th	(1) 13th	
	(4) Interview for promotion	15th		
	(5) Turned down for promotion	19th		31
	(6) Son lost £10 of his money	19th	(2) 20th	
			(3) 22nd	
			(4) 24th	
			(5) 30th	
			(6) 31st	
17	(1) Threatened with eviction	2nd	(1) 1st	
	(2) Told he had liver disease by GP	2nd	(2) 2nd	
	(3) Eviction notice withdrawn	5th	(3) 5th	13
	(4) Hospital outpatient attendance for liver disease		(4) 6th	
		9th	(5) 9th	
			(6) 11th	
20	(1) Severe angina requiring hospital attention	5th	(1) 8th	
	(2) Admitted to Maudsley Hospital (depressive illness)	6th		
	(3) Severe angina	7th		
	(4) Ward social/anniversary of wife's death	8th		22
	(5) Discharge from Maudsley Hospital	11th		
	(6) Readmission to Maudsley Hospital	17th		
	(7) Discharge from Maudsley Hospital	20th		
22	(1) Closest friend went on holiday	9th	(1) 9th	13

The events fell into four main groups. First *personal interaction* (an event involving a disturbance in an emotional relationship which seemed to the doctor and patient an important one (approximately 33 per cent of the events). Secondly *work* events which involved a change or possible change in the patient's working life (approximately 33 per cent of events). *Health* events which involved a health change in the subject or in members of his household of sufficient severity to require hospital attention (approximately 20 per cent of events). Finally, *residential* change in events which involved a change or possible change of residence (approximately 13 per cent of events).

From inspection of Table 15.1 a temporal relationship between events and relapse appears likely at least in some patients. In patients Nos. 1, 6, 7, 10, 15, 17 and 22 episodes of relapse followed events in the patients' lives either in the same week or following two weeks. In the remaining patients this did not seem to be the case; further events occurred without relapse following. Taking the patients as a whole, i.e., the 22 patients, no significant correlation was found between number of events patients experienced and frequency of relapse. It is difficult to assess statistically the importance that an event contributes to a relapse for the practical reason that throughout the study events are freely occurring, and a comparison of the probability of relapse under conditions where events can freely occur and when they cannot is, of course, impossible. Thus, although in seven patients the impression was of a relationship between events and subsequent relapse no statistical relationship was established.

The Brown and Birley questionnaire used in this study has in the past only been used in a retrospective manner. Because of the potential importance of this tool it was thought useful for comparison to record the percentage of alcoholic patients who experienced events of the Brown and Birley type and compare them with the percentage of Brown and Birley subjects in study who experienced such events. This is shown in Table 15.2.

Discussion

It should be mentioned at the outset that because of the small numbers in this study conclusions must be tentative. The study did have the advantage, however, of being prospective, and care being taken to date the onset of events and relapses accurately. The study was part of a larger study (Hore, 1971) which showed in general that relapse in the alcoholic undergoing treatment as an outpatient is frequent, and usually appears suddenly without a previous build up in anxiety, depression or craving. In some patients, as stated above, relapse appears to occur as a result of events in the patients' lives, although no statistical relationship between events and relapse was established. It is of interest that whilst events of the personal interaction type

102

Table 15.2
Comparison of the percentage of patients in this study experiencing
BB type events with schizophrenic patients and controls in
Brown and Birley's study

	Average percentage of patients experiencing events in a 3-week period		
	Independent	Possibly independent	Both
BB control population	14.5	5.3	19.5
Schizophrenics*	12.0	10.2	22.6
Alcoholics in this study	14.7	8.8	22.1

* These figures are the average for the 3-week periods of this study excluding the 3 weeks before schizophrenic breakdown, when they showed a considerable increase.

were of first importance, work events were of equal importance and health events only slightly less. The types of events seen in alcoholics' lives do not seem on inspection to differ from those occurring in non-alcoholics and their frequency of occurrence resembles that of a control and schizophrenic population using the same method of data recording (Table 15.2). This similarity using the Brown and Birley questionnaire when it is used prospectively and retrospectively gives some weight to the validity of the questionnaire. It might be important to distinguish those alcoholics who respond to events by relapse ('event sensitive') from those who do not ('non-event sensitive'). It was not possible with the limited numbers in this study to see any clear factors which separated the two however; this might form the aim of a larger study. If it was possible to become aware of a particular alcoholic's areas of psychological vulnerability, especially in the stage of alcoholism before physical dependency existed, the alcoholic might learn ways of coping other than drinking alcohol.

16 Aversion therapy and attitude change in the treatment of alcoholism*

W. FALKOWSKI

Summary

Pilot work is described which was directed toward design of a behavioural treatment for alcoholism, and a treatment based on social-psychological approaches to attitude change. The feasibility of the two methods and the use of parallel outcome methods was explored in a small preliminary trial.

Introduction

The purpose of this study was to develop and pilot two contrasting treatment methods, with each related to a particular theoretical model. The first approach was a package of aversion therapies based on specific aspects of learning theory; the second approach (attitude change) had its basis in certain theoretical aspects of social psychology, with special note here being made of the possible therapeutic applications of cognitive dissonance.

Literature review

The relevant literature is critically reviewed. As regards the literature on aversion therapy for alcoholism, it is concluded that firm evidence for the efficacy of any of the methods which have up to now been reported is still lacking. Research has often been methodologically poor and has notably lacked controls. The patient–therapist relationship in alcoholism aversion treatment remains largely unexplored, despite its probable importance. The emotional response generated during the aversive conditioning is worthy of attention, and the cognitive effect of aversive conditioning for alcoholism has also been neglected. Most surprisingly, in none of the studies noted in this review was there reported any systematic attempt to measure in what proportion of subjects, and to what degree, was the hoped-for aversion

---

* Synopsis of an unpublished dissertation of the same title by W. Falkowski which was submitted successfully in 1970 to the University of London in part fulfilment of requirements for the degree of M. Phil.

actually induced. Relationship between degree of aversion (however measured) and subsequent sobriety remains, therefore, a very open question; the relationship may not be linear. Little has been done to exploit physiological measures.

The relevant general literature on attitude formation and attitude change is then discussed, and it is concluded that there is a considerable volume of evidence in favour of prediction (based on cognitive-dissanance theory) of an immense incentive-attitude change relationship, i.e. in simple terms, the bigger the demand for change and the confrontation, the less likely that attitude will actually shift. It is further concluded that active participation in role-playing is a more potent change mechanism than putting the subject in the passive position of simply being receiver of given information. The literature on fear-arousal is considered and the relationship between the effectiveness of such communication and the individual's ability to cope with anxiety is examined; interpretation of this body of writing is still to a degree problematical but note is taken of the apparent finding that high fear communications are likely to be particularly ineffective on patients who are highly and chronically anxious.

Design of two theoretically-based treatments

1 *Aversion conditioning procedures:* (a) The 'drinking' stimuli where projected slides depicting 'drinking' situations, (b) 'drinking alcohol' in fantasy, and (c) experience of smell and taste of several common beverages. The aversive stimulus was electric shock of variable intensity and duration, adjusted for each individual so as to be highly unpleasant, but not intolerable. Positive reinforcement was given by social-verbal approach on patients selecting non-alcoholic drink on avoidance trials. Paradigms were set up for 'punishment', 'escape', and 'avoidance' learning.

2 *Attitude modification procedures.* The treatment was in three phases. (a) Presentation of a hierarchy of statements about alcohol to the patient, to which he was required to express agreement or disagreement; as treatment proceeded he was gradually exposed to questions which might more and more tax his motivation; any question which excited a pro-alcohol response was temporarily withdrawn. (b) Role-playing sessions involving fear arousal: the sessions consisted of the patient projecting himself in fantasy into the future and recounting to the therapist the misfortunes which might have resulted from his drinking. (c) Role-playing self-persuasion using a tape recorder: in a final session the subject was asked to make as persuasive a recording as possible of his personal reasons for giving up drink.

A pilot controlled trial

Four patients were randomly allocated to each of a control (milieu) group, an aversion group and an attitude change group. Patients in the latter two groups each received a total of 15 individual sessions lasting 30–45 minutes. Outcome measures included sematic differential measures of attitude toward drink, measures of patient therapist relationship, of mood change during treatment, while for follow-up period after discharge ($4\frac{1}{2}$–12 months) assessment was made of abstinence, work record and marital adjustment.

This investigation was conceived of simply as exploratory and the between-group results are obviously seen as of much lesser importance than what was learnt regarding development of techniques and measurements. On the basis of the lessons learnt, a detailed research schedule is finally proposed as blue-print for a larger and more definitive study.

In the definitive study the developed questionnaire was filled out as a self-completion inventory by a sample of 390 alcoholic subjects who were members of Alcoholics Anonymous or a private practice support group (Renaissance Group). Problems of sampling and response bias are discussed. Central hypotheses were tested by (1) comparing on multiple dimensions the characteristics of the subgroup who had been 'occupationally exposed' (by occupational definition) during the ten years prior to onset of alcoholism, with the remainder; (2) similar comparison with sample split by presence or absence of 'occupational sub-factors'.

Methodological difficulties are discussed at length, and the author sees this work more as concerned with development of a theoretical framework for future and more rigorous researches than its allowing anything approaching firm conclusions. The tentative conclusion would, however, be that the true importance of occupation in the genesis of alcoholism may be much smaller than 'common sense' would propose.

17   A controlled trial of alcohol dependence employing 'maximum' and 'minimum' therapeutic modalities*

JIM ORFORD and THE PROJECT TEAM

Summary

A short preliminary account is given of a controlled trial in which 100 married male alcoholics were randomised between a 'maximum' and 'minimum' treatment régime.

Introduction

We report here simply on the design of a clinical trial. This paper thus deals with 'research in progress' rather than reporting any results and the inclusion of such a note requires some justification − a report without results may seem to have something of *Hamlet* without the last act. Our reason for including an account of this study's methodology at what might seem a premature stage is the belief that methodology and research design are in themselves at times worth discussion and critical appraisal.

This trial has been designed as a test of a crucial question concerning the efficacy of the conventional package which constitutes the essence of alcoholism treatment in many parts of the world today. Is the reported 'success' rate obtained by this treatment approach greater than the 'spontaneous' remission rate? Are patients with good treatment prognosis simply those who have good 'spontaneous' remission characteristics?

The design of any trial which is to resolve this key question presents difficulties. It is neither ethical nor practical to set up a control 'placebo' group analogous to that employed in a conventional drug trial. The chosen strategy has been to take the analogy of dose–response testing. If a drug given in high

---

* An account written for this volume of a controlled trial, the results of which are now in the process of final analysis. The research team consisted of Jim Orford (psychologist); Stella Egert, Sally Guthrie, Ann Hawker, Celia Hensman, Edna Oppenheim (research social workers); Griffith Edwards and Martin Mitcheson (psychiatrists). A. N. Oppenheim advised on research planning.

dose is no more potent than the substance given in a lower dose, then unless it is to be argued that the high dose is super-maximal, it may fairly be concluded that the drug is probably lacking in potency; at the very least it may be concluded that there is no routine practical advantage in giving the higher dose.

Case selection

One hundred married male alcoholics consecutively attending the Maudsley Hospital after full assessment, but otherwise unselected allocated to one or other treatment group by randomisation.

Initial assessments

Initial assessments were made at the outpatient clinic. During the course of an approximately three and one half hour session full structured histories were taken independently from husband and wife; on the husband a mental state and physical examination were performed and laboratory testing arranged; a variety of specially designed attitude scales were administered to assess motivation towards abstinence and aspects of family functioning; observation was made of husband/wife interaction in a structured interview situation.

Treatment modalities

1 *Maximum régime*

Each patient was under the continuing care of one particular psychiatrist, who would initially attempt outpatient treatment; the package included counselling or psychotherapy with or without aversive drugs as indicated and attention to physical health. The goal was total abstinence and if there was not speedy response to OP care the patient was admitted to a specialised group-therapy oriented inpatient alcoholism unit. In parallel to this psychiatric care, an individual social worker was allocated to the wife of each patient; the social worker's role was to work with the wife (and the family) at reality and at dynamic levels; home visits were frequently made, and if the patient himself broke contact with the clinic, the social worker would often still be able to maintain useful contact with the wife. Husbands were offered introduction to Alcoholics Anonymous and wives to Al-Anon.

2 *Minimum régime*

Immediately following the initial assessment, a joint counselling session was held with husband and wife. They were informed of the diagnosis of alcoholism and it was stressed that the implication of this diagnosis was that the husband had now to aim at total abstinence. They were told that reaching the goal was the husband's responsibility and only he could make the personal decision as to whether he did or did not in future drink. In the event of his developing withdrawal symptoms he was advised to contact his general practitioner. Advice was also given in other life areas. No subsequent hospital contact was offered but it was explained (see below) that someone would visit the wife for monthly information.

Follow up

All patients were followed up for 12 months after intake. For both groups, detailed monthly information was obtained by the research social worker from the spouse; for the treatment group, monthly assessments were also obtained by the doctor from the patient. At the end of 12 months, families in both groups were re-assessed in detail on the basis of lengthy interviews with both husband and wife. Multiple outcome measures were used concerning family adjustment and other aspects of social functioning, as well as drinking behaviour.

Ethical safeguards

If one of the monthly reports which the research social workers obtained from a 'minimum' régime wife suggested a seriously deteriorating position, the social worker might call an immediate staff conference to discuss crossing the family over to 'maximum' régime. In the event it was necessary to cross over two out of the 50 'minimum' régime families in this way; the minimum régime families had of course open possibility of contact with their family doctor, and had the option of seeking specialised referral elsewhere.

Analysis strategy

Follow-up to 12 months has been completed and an analysis is now in progress which will seek (1) to compare groups on multiple outcome variables; (2) to determine correlations between outcomes and multiple descriptive variables and attitude measurements (with particular reference to family functioning); (3) to examine certain methodological problems, e.g., the relation between husbands' and wives' reports.

109

18 Appraisal

To determine whether a particular bottle of blue medicine is good for bronchitis is a reasonably simple affair. The double-blind controlled trial has its pitfalls, but give or take a little it can establish whether a medicine is effective in the treatment of a particular medical condition. It might therefore be hoped that a ready investigatory tool is at hand to determine whether a given approach to alcoholism is effective.

There would certainly be agreement that simple uncontrolled observation of a case series can with alcoholism take one so far but no further. The finding, for instance, that patients who go to Alcoholics Anonymous have a better outcome could mean that AA is an effective treatment, or might only indicate that patients who are motivated and who in any case have a favourable outlook, then as token of their good intent join AA. AA becomes, as it were, consequence rather than cause. To raise such an alternative explanation is sometimes mere hair splitting, but here the alternative explanation seems credible, and cannot lightly be dismissed. For the alcoholism researcher to reach for the methods of the controlled trial is, in these circumstances, the seemingly obvious research strategy.

That researcher had best however reach with some caution. A treatment tool which is aptly designed for assessing the worth of blue medicine in the treatment of a relatively definable medical condition can provide a basic model for investigation of more complex medico-social problems, but the investigator will be led into naive disasters if he supposes that the tool requires no rejigging. Satisfactorily to mount a controlled trial on a multi-dimensional condition such as alcoholism must involve conceptual clarity of design, where all the invitations are to complexity, solution of a range of extremely difficult methodological problems, painstaking and determined fieldwork, and finally an approach to data analysis which consistently aims toward the greatest possible simplicity.

Some of the reasons for believing that the alcoholism controlled trial brings a quite different level of complexity than the blue medicine investigation which epitomises the parentage of this scientific art form, might then be listed as follows:

1 *The validity of data.* Alcoholism treatment research by-and-large will utilise as its data simply what people say, rather than anything more concrete. The informant is the patient himself (who may be expected by no means

110

always to give an accurate picture), or use is made of the so-called independent informant, e.g., the spouse. Little work has been done on the biases which may distort that so-called independent report. Research stating that results were 'confirmed by an independent informant in every case', must inevitably homogenise disparate and contradictory statements. Harder data such as drunkenness arrest or hospitalisation subsequent to treatment may indeed also be collected, but each sets its own problems in interpretation.

2 *Determining what is to be measured.* Alcoholism is a condition of uncertain pathology and multiple social and medical manifestations. The decision therefore as to what is to be measured sets problems: the invitation is toward a broad sweep and measurement (with uncertain measuring instruments) of everything within reach. Later comes the headache of analysis. Drinking behaviour itself may appear appealing as the commonsensical crux of the matter, but accurate description of quantity, frequency, and variability of drinking behaviour, is no easy matter. How is a patient who over the course of a year engages in one month's chaotic drinking to be compared against the subject who over 12 months drinks heavily over 12 weekends? The possible patterns of drinking (and consequent social disabilities) are legion, and any simple rule-of-thumb categorisation can by the arbitrary choice of categories radically effect the results.

3 *The measurement of change.* To be able to measure change assumes knowledge of the base-line from which change is to take place. If follow-up is to be for the 12 months after treatment, then presumably the base-line must be the 12 months prior to treatment, and this involves collection of data the validity of which will be quite uncertainly influenced by lapse of memory and retrospective falsification.

4 *Sampling problems and comparability of groups.* Trials are at their simplest when the nature of the condition being treated readily allows definition of a homogeneous population by setting up a few criteria for 'inclusion' and 'exclusion', and where randomisation between groups can therefore be expected to provide well matched sub-samples. Matching by such randomisation is not nearly so certain when the patient population is heterogenous in regard to all manner of variables which may well relate to treatment outcome. The larger the groups presumably so much the better, but even with large groups we may guess that there remains fairly high probability of some aberrance in matching. How large is large?

5 *Holding all else constant.* The classic model of the controlled trial assumes that the efficacy of two treatments can be compared because the two patient groups are otherwise not subjected to any treatment influence over the trial period, or are submitted to identical background treatment influences, e.g., 'general nursing care'. With alcoholism the trial period has usually been

111

of 12 months or longer duration: over such a spell it is not possible to control extraneous treatment happenings or life events (the relevance of Hore's paper becomes obvious) – one patient may meet up with an interested general practitioner, another patient's house may burn down. The investigator must rest on the hope that on average the same chance good-fortune and catastrophe will befall the two patient groups equally, an assumption which usually rests on hope rather than being supported by any demonstration. Hope will certainly be ill-founded if there is a reason for the two treatment modalities being in some manner differentially associated with 'extraneous' influences, e.g., when the patients in one group are more interesting to the staff and the 'general nursing care' which they receive is of a different kind and quantity than the other group, or when the two modalities in any way excite differential (compensatory) help-seeking activity by the two patient groups.

6 *Incomplete follow-up.* With the original blue-medicine version of the art-form it would generally be thought shameful if over the four week trial period 20 per cent of patients were lost to the final observation. If an alcoholism trial runs for a 12 month period it is quite to be expected that 20 per cent of patients will be lost to the final follow-up. If these patients are those who have fared less well, the 80 per cent of either group will give a spuriously optimistic picture of treatment success. So far as between-group comparisons are concerned this does not matter provided again that there is no likelihood of a differential bias. That two different treatment approaches should result in different types and patterns of contact breaking would however seem not inconceivable.

7 *Double-blind.* A feature of the classical trial design is that neither patient nor observer should know which treatment is being given. With alcoholism investigations both these conditions have usually remained quite starkly unmet: the hypnosis trial and IP/OP trial reported in this book both fail in this regard, and only the metronidazole trial fulfils the demand. Furthermore, in most published research it appears to be a member of the therapeutic team who collects the follow-up data. In terms of the cannons of the blue-medicine trial, it could be said that most work on alcoholism treatment ignores the most fundamental rules of the game.

To dismiss most of the above points as just petty quibbling about tiny bits of possible variance would be the comfortable way of dealing with the critics. The temptation is to retreat to the fond hope that all will come right in the wash, that given a bit of luck all the errors will balance out, and the truth will come through. The critics cannot really however be so lightly put down: there may indeed be so many sources of small or larger error around, and (most importantly) so many possibilities of that error being non-random with systematic bias related to treatment modality, that false 'truths' will come through, or real truths be concealed. For alcoholism treatment studies the controlled trial is not the easy cure-all which it might have been hoped.

An appraisal of the papers presented in this part of the book would in essence seem to point up the need for further investment in two general lines of development. The first would be the painstaking refinement of all matters related to the techniques of investigating treatment efficacy, and in this regard we should not be mesmerised into believing that the large-scale controlled trial is the only possible art-form. More thought should be given to alternative strategies such as the detailed investigation of small groups (or single cases), cast much more in the terms of experimental manipulation of this or that closely defined behavioural variable. The second line of investment should be the design of new treatment methods which rationally apply behavioural or social-psychological techniques. The pilot investigation which Falkowski reports provides an example of the sort of groundwork which is much needed.

Part IV The community

19 Alcoholics Anonymous: the anatomy of a self help group*

GRIFFITH EDWARDS, CELIA HENSMAN, ANN HAWKER and
VALERIE WILLIAMSON

Summary

A self-completion inventory was filled by 306 AA members who attended
meetings in London during the course of one week. Details are given of
demographic social and personality characteristics; hospital treatment
experience; AA involvement; drinking history and length of sobriety;
complications and associations of drinking. It is argued that AA, despite its
overt open door policy, covertly 'selects' by offering a strongly characterised
'ideal' member, with whom not all potential members will be able to identify.
AA is as much a supportive organisation for the chronic relapsing subject as
it is a treatment organisation.

Introduction

Surprisingly little is known about who goes to Alcoholics Anonymous in this
country. In England, the only attempt to collect descriptive data on an AA
population was that carried out by Cooper and Maule (1962). A more recent
American report written by an AA member, Bill C. (1965), has given a fuller
and probably more accurate account of who goes to AA than previously
available for the USA, but this study was of alcoholics showing some
regularity of attendance at meetings, rather than of the total AA population.
Confident interpretation of the results of much previous work is to an extent
hampered by the uncertain nature of the sampling.

---

* A condensed version of a paper of the same title which originally appeared
in *Social Psychiatry,* vol. 1, 1967, pp. 195–204.

Method

Design of questionnaire

The schedule contained 15 items on drinking history and AA attendance, 22 items on complications of excessive drinking, and 23 demographic and social items. The 12 questions of the short scale of the Maudsley Personality Inventory (Eysenck 1959) were also included. Social stability, both at present and at the time of joining AA, was rated on a five-point scale derived from Straus and Bacon (1951). Social class was determined on the basis of occupation using the Registrar General's Classification of Occupation (General Register Office, 1960).

Distribution and collection of questionnaires

Batches of questionnaires were sent to the group secretary of each meeting for use at all meetings held in London during one week of 1964. Secretaries were asked to ensure that every member present at any meeting completed a questionnaire, unless one had been filled in at an earlier meeting in the same week. The plan adopted was that, at the close of the meeting, the secretary should collect the completed forms and send them to the research office, rather than permitting members to take the questionnaires home (with the attendant uncertainties of individual co-operation).

Results

Co-operation

Co-operation was obtained with 40 (89 per cent) of the 45 groups which should have held meetings during the week of the study. As a result of the approach to individual AA members coming to each meeting by the group's own secretary, the number of members of any group failing to complete a questionnaire was very small; the precise figure could not, however, be determined. A total of 306 completed questionnaires was returned.

Data

(The notation ± will be used throughout to indicate 95 per cent confidence limits on the mean).
1   *Sex.* Of the 306 members 248 (81 per cent) were men and 58 (19 per cent) were women.
2   *Age.* The mean age was 45.7 ± 1.7 for men, 45.6 ± 2.1 for women. Four per cent were aged 20–29, and 22, 42, 24, 7 and 1 per cent were in successive

ten year age-groups up to 70–79.

3   *Marital status*. Details of present marital status are set out in Table 19.1.

Table 19.1

Marital status: percentage of subjects in each category

Marital status	Men n = 248	Women n = 58	Total n = 306
Single	18	26	19
Married	60	46	58
Separated	12	11	12
Divorced	8	8	8
Widowed	2	9	3

4   *Social class*. Enquiry was made into both 'present' and 'best' social class; the analysis is given in Table 19.2.

Table 19.2

Present social class and best social class: percentage of members in each category

	I	II	III	IV	V	Not categorised
Total: present	9	26	50	10	4	1
best	12	32	45	9	1	1

5   *Social stability*. Data is given in Table 19.3.

6   *Personality*. Findings on the present group, on Eysenck's original standardisation sample and on a normal population surveyed in London (Hare and Shaw, 1965) are given in Table 19.4. The AA population have a significantly higher mean N score (neuroticism) than Eysenck's standardisation group ($P < .01$) and although information was not given by Hare and Shaw on the standard deviation of the N score of their population, it appears probable that here too the AA group has a significantly higher N score. The mean E score (extraversion) of AA members resembles that of a normal population.

117

Table 19.3
Social stability score (Straus and Bacon scale) of AA and
two hospital samples. Means and 95% confidence limits on means

Study	Type of population		Number	Mean SS score
AA: time of joining	Male		217	2.5 ± 0.2
	Female		44	2.3 ± 0.4
	Total		261	2.5 ± 0.2
AA: time of enquiry	Male	AA	238	2.5 ± 0.2
	Female		51	2.2 ± 0.4
	Total		289	2.4 ± 0.2
Davies et al. (1956)	Hospital		39	1.5 ± 0.5
Edwards (1966)	Hospital		40	2.4

Table 19.4
Scores of AA members and normal populations on N (neuroticism)
and E (extraversion) scales of short form of Maudsley personality
inventory. Means and 95% confidence limits on means

Population	Sample size	Mean N	Mean E	% Scoring N 10, 11, 12 (extreme)
AA male	248	8.82 ± .43	7.32 ± .38	58.9
AA female	58	7.46 ± .95	8.67 ± .70	32.8
AA total	306	8.59 ± .40	7.57 ± .34	53.9
Eysenck's normals	1600	6.15 ± .17	7.96 ± .15	–
London:				
new suburb male	496	4.64	6.93	9.2
female	431	4.73	7.27	15.5
old suburb male	519	5.82	6.78	12.1
female	494	5.08	6.76	15.4

7 *Age at which drinking first became a problem.* For men the mean age given was 28.5 ± 1.2, for women 33.9 ± 2.2 years (P < 0.05).

8 *Hospital treatment for alcoholism.* Both among the men and among the women 60 per cent had received inpatient treatment for alcoholism at least once and respectively there was some overlap between those who had

received inpatient and outpatient care: 33 per cent of both men and women had received neither.

9   *Duration of AA membership.* Distributions are given in Table 19.5. The mean duration was 50 ± 5.8 months for men, 38 ± 9.3 months for women.

Table 19.5
Duration of AA membership in years; distribution in percentages

Duration	Men n = 241	Women n = 55
0– 6 months	22	16
7–12 months	6	7
— 2 years	13	23
— 4 years	17	24
— 6 years	15	16
— 8 years	11	2
—10 years	8	9
10+ years	8	2

10   *Frequency of AA attendance.* Subjects were asked which of the following statements described their pattern of attendance most closely:

	Percentage
'Most nights'	20
'At least once in most weeks'	73
'At least once in most months'	3
'Just dropping in occasionally'	4

There was no difference in distribution between men and women.

11   *Duration of sobriety.* The question asked was 'How long is it since you last had a drink?' Forty two per cent of members had been sober for only six months or less, but the maximum period was almost 15 years. The mean duration was 30.3 ± 4.1 months for men, 21.9 ± 7.8 months for women.

12   *Number of 'slips' since joining AA.* Forty three per cent of 293 subjects said that they had not 'slipped' by their own definition since joining AA: 29 per cent had slipped once or twice, 10 per cent had slipped three to four times and 18 per cent had slipped five or more times. Subjects with less than one month's membership were excluded from the analysis. There was no difference in distribution between men and women.

13   *Complications and accompaniments of excessive drinking.* In table 19.6, which gives the actual wording of the questions, the percentage of subjects answering 'yes' to a selection of the original 23 questions is set out. The right-hand column indicates which phenomena showed a significant between-sex difference.

Table 19.6

Incidence of complications and accompaniments of excessive drinking.
(Significance of between-sex differences: ** P<0.01, * P<0.05)

	Men		Women	
	n	%	n	%
Had 'blackouts' (patches of completely blank memory) through drinking	248	95	57	91
Had severe morning shakes	248	84	58	72
** lost a job because of drinking	247	63	56	43
* Had DTs – that is, shaky, confused and seeing things	246	59	54	43
* Been arrested for being drunk	244	49	58	29
** Been in a serious fight because of drinking	247	40	57	19
Broken up a marriage because of drinking	239	35	57	28
** Attempted suicide because of drinking	244	26	57	47
Been in prison because of drinking	246	22	58	12
Had a stomach or duodenal ulcer	246	19	58	21
Been convicted of drunken driving	244	16	56	7
Been arrested for being drunk 5 or more times	241	15	56	9

Discussion

The results

1   *Demographic factors.* A general picture of Alcoholics Anonymous in London can now be sketched. This is an organisation in which male exceeds female membership by four to one. AA draws its greatest strength from those who are middle-aged and the social class of its members is preponderantly class III or above. Almost 60 per cent of members are married and living with

spouse, and social stability, as measured on a derivation of the Straus-Bacon scale, shows that AA is far from being a society of the drifting.

The extent to which these demographic data convey a 'true' picture of alcoholism may be questioned, as opposed to their giving a picture distorted by selection processes inherent in AA affiliation. The 'true' picture of alcoholism in any society – that picture which is undistorted by the idiosyncratic sampling bias of any particular treatment agency – is almost impossible to obtain. What can be claimed with certainty is that the unskilled labourer is as unlikely to be found in AA as in the alcoholism unit – despite his often being found before the magistrate. The explanation is either the unlikely one that alcoholism is rare in social class V, or that AA, like the hospitals, operates a powerful selection process.

2 *Personality.* The conclusion may probably be drawn that neuroticism and extraversion fail to differentiate AA from hospital alcoholics. The finding that the mean E score of AA members is not significantly greater than that of a normal population does something to contradict the idea that AA is particularly attractive to the more roistering and exhibitionistic individual.

3 *Age at which drinking first became a problem.* Whatever the basis on which each subject is making a judgement, the fact emerges that men see their drinking problem as having arisen at an earlier age on average than do women. For the drinking problem first to have arisen in an AA member after the age of 50 is rare – only 2.6 per cent of membership had this late onset. This finding provides an interesting parallel to the classical belief that the first onset of neurotic symptoms is seldom in middle age.

4 *Hospital treatment for alcoholism.* The failure of either the majority of demographic or the E and N scores to differentiate AA from reported hospital series becomes more explicable: to a large extent the two populations overlap. This overlap is, no doubt, partly a reflection of the good relationship which exists in London between AA and doctors. To suggest that AA is increasingly serving as an aftercare – and perhaps pre-care – organisation, rather than playing its original and more autonomous role, is in no way to lower its valuation.

5 *Duration of AA membership.* The mean duration of AA membership was over four years, and the picture which comes from Table 19.5 is of an organisation with a large percentage of faithful hard-core members, and a smaller component of transients, most of whom drop out after about six months. Who are these transient attenders? A guess is that they are not only alcoholics who are lost to AA because of their immediate relapse or insincerity of intention, but include many who find it impossible to identify with the AA image. The present results do seem to underline the fact that a considerable number of alcoholics, after a more or less brief attendance at

meetings, find that AA is not to their liking and cannot help them.

6 *Frequency and regularity of AA attendance.* AA seems to consist largely of members who are energetic in their attendance. Someone who goes to AA tends typically to go regularly and often and for a long time.

7 *Duration of sobriety and number of slips.* The most important finding as regards duration of sobriety is that 42 per cent of members had been sober for no longer than six months. This fact must be set against there being only 21 per cent of members who have been in AA for six months or less – the explanation of a considerable proportion having had only a short period of sobriety is not therefore the loading by new members. The average of 28.8 months sobriety for the group as a whole is a reflection of the skewed distribution with its long upper tail. The findings on the number of slips which members have experienced since joining AA serves further to bring out the point that AA is as much a society of alcoholics who are having difficulty in remaining sober as it is one in which they are staying off drink. This interpretation however must not be pushed too far, for although it is evident that more than half the members have slipped since joining AA and 18 per cent more than five times, 43 per cent of members have remained completely sober.

The total picture which comes from these results suggests that an accurate assessment of AA's achievements requires rather a different emphasis from that usually given. AA is of course in part a 'treatment' organisation achieving 'cure' or 'arrest', and it is these therapeutic successes which have given it prestige. This emphasis has inevitably led to the neglect of a less dramatic but perhaps more important and more unique achievement: AA has created a supportive organisation which accepts and continues to tolerate the relapsing alcoholic who has little ability to maintain long-term sobriety. A question deserving investigation is the ability of AA to modify the severity of the 'slip' without preventing it. AA may assist a man in cutting short the drinking bout, with less damage done than there would have been if AA had not helped. A count of 'slips' which ignores their severity cannot give the complete picture.

8 *Complications and accompaniments of excessive drinking.* If a subject's having suffered from 'severe morning shakes' can be taken as evidence of pharmacological dependence on alcohol then 82 per cent of members were chemically dependent. The preponderence amongst AA members of those syndromes which imply an element of 'addiction' must again be seen as something bearing on the particular stereotype of 'the alcoholic' which figures in AA's teaching. The man or woman who has not experienced 'loss of control' is going to find identification difficult. It is widely held in AA that an alcoholic must 'experience rock bottom' before being able to accept help and

the severe damage shown in the present analysis to have been suffered by so many AA members is, no doubt, the group experience which forms the basis of the group's assertion. And again this formulation of the 'ideal' may be suspected of influencing the selection process: the problem drinker who cannot himself catalogue a series of disastrous experiences may have difficulty in identifying.

Final conclusion

A postulate which has been used repeatedly in interpreting the findings of this study is that AA *selects* – that, despite the declared policy of having no bar to membership, there are inevitable covert and dynamic selection processes at work. The task of selection, which in orthodox and 'led-group' therapy is an important responsibility borne by the therapist, is in AA somehow carried out by the group itself. Selection is not effected by showing the nonconforming member the door, but by AA establishing norms of what the good AA member is to be. If the newcomer deviates too far from these norms, he will find identification very difficult and is then unlikely to be seen at many meetings.

Identification is the very essence of the affiliation process. The role played by the sponsor may sometimes be important, but can be exaggerated: identification is not with any one established member so much as with fragments of a whole series of life histories which are synthesised into identification with the group ideal. Identification assumes particular importance in the leaderless group which must have a clear and firmly-established picture of the ideal member. Although this picture may partly be based on the statistical norm, it derives also in some measure from the group's fantasy and wishfulfilment.

The present report, as has already been stressed, is a study of Alcoholics Anonymous in one particular city; but this world-wide organisation has so much to tell research workers that it is bound increasingly to attract investigation. Research will produce new facts and will force fresh interpretations, but if the present study is any guide, growth of understanding will only enhance admiration.

20 In place of Skid Row: the first three years of the Rathcoole Experiment, May 1966 – May 1969*

TIMOTHY COOK and BENNO POLLAK

Summary

The development of a ten bedded rehabilitation centre for male Skid Row alcoholics is described. Over the course it evolved from a fairly conventional and unsuccessful hostel into an effective therapeutic community: the trial-and-error learning and the practical strategems which underlay that evolution are analysed in detail. Problems certainly still remain, but lessons have been learnt which perhaps bear on the planning of future rehabilitation services and which also perhaps give some hint as to how prevention might be tackled.

Introduction

Rathcoole House is a late Victorian mansion situated in South London. A voluntary committee of professional workers in the field of alcoholism opened the house in May 1966 as an experiment in the rehabilitation of the male habitual drunkenness offender. It was guaranteed financially for its first two years by the Carnegie Trust, and for a further two years by the Home Office. It was hoped that the men would go out to work each day, returning to normal home comforts in the evening, though work was not obligatory. The house accommodated ten men and, when working, each would contribute £4.10s.0d. per week towards his rent; when not in work, the rent would be met by the Ministry of Social Security. The staff initially consisted of a resident warden, assistant warden and Community Service volunteer, with a non-resident cook and cleaner.

The possible significance of the Rathcoole experiment has, in England, been

---

* An abridgement of a report of the same title which originally appeared as No. 4 in the series of NACRO papers and reprints (published in 1970 by National Association for Care and Rehabilitation of Offenders, 125 Kennington Park Road, London, SE11).

enhanced by section 91 of the 1967 Criminal Justice Act. In effect, this states that imprisonment for drunkenness will be abolished provided 'suitable alternatives' can be established; this section will only be implemented when the Home Secretary is satisfied that such suitable alternatives do, in fact, exist.

It should be made very clear that the whole project was seen as an experiment, a venture which – with the collection of data on the residents and their life in the house – would lead, by trial and error, towards the development of new ideas. The purpose of the experiment was to generate ideas and to test their practicality. Exploration continues and there are still many unanswered questions, for Rathcoole is certainly not a final answer. Despite our limited knowledge, we nonetheless had some preconceptions and the history of the house so far has largely been one of the abandonment of preconceptions.

In the first year the men were helped by little other than simple supportive measures, but these seemed to produce only very limited success. However, the fact that some of our preconceptions had already been disproved led us to believe that we should not, once again, reject the men as being 'impossible to help' but look at the system of help we were offering, and whether it was really appropriate to their needs. One factor in particular encouraged in us the view that there was a greater potential amongst the men than, previously, we had been prepared to admit. This was in their attitude to work. We had anticipated the men being work shy and malingerers, and often incapable of work, but without exception the men were almost over-enthusiastic to obtain work. The staff dissuaded men from starting work too soon rather than persuaded them to look for work. Another interesting and unexpected indication of hope was the men's early morning routine. From the beginning they showed a willingness to get themselves up, cook their own breakfast and get themselves off to work. This was in marked contrast to the warden's previous experience in a house for non-alcoholic ex-offenders.

In essence, the second year was one in which we moved away from simple supportive measures to trying to establish a real therapeutic community. This, naturally, was a difficult year which made considerable demands upon both the staff and the residents.

The third year was both a consolidation of and development of the therapeutic community ideas, only tenuously established during the second year. The house, however, is at all times experimental and the present phase is by no means to be regarded as closed and complete. Nothing of what follows is intended to suggest that problems now do not occur. They do – every day.

We would now like to examine these three phases in more detail.

1   Admission policy

Potential residents have always been referred to us from a variety of sources and always on a voluntary basis. The primary sources of referral are prison, probation and after-care service, hospitals, the reception centre, Alcoholics Anonymous, and church missions. To some extent, whom we select is determined by who is referred to us. The nature and the quality of the referral can vary enormously. It is certainly true to say that over the three years, the general quality of referrals has improved, which reflects not only a greater seriousness on the part of those referring, but also an increased ability on the part of both residents and staff at Rathcoole to communicate to others what the house really stands for.

In principle, every man who is referred is seen by the staff and rarely is a man rejected without at least one interview. Over the three years, however, the method of selection has changed enormously. Initially, the staff interviewed the applicant and, if selected, introduced him to the other residents. It was gradually realised, however, that while such a system of selection was simple and authoritative, it did have certain disadvantages. First, in the London Skid Row culture, many of the men already knew each other, and often, information about a man which might have influenced the selection only later came to the knowledge of the staff. It was felt that we should make better use both of the men's specific knowledge of each other, and also of their general understanding of the alcoholic. Secondly, when staff selected the residents and made the inevitable mistakes, they were then used as scapegoats by the men for the difficulties that resulted. This only served to increase staff–resident division making it more difficult to create any sense of community. Thirdly, the selection procedure discouraged resident involvement in the house which we felt it essential to develop.

At the beginning of the second year, we introduced the idea at a house meeting that the residents should be given an opportunity to vote on a man's entry into the house. Initially, the idea was rejected – the residents argued that they would not sit in judgement on a fellow-alcoholic. Eventually it was agreed that the men would at least try to operate a system whereby they had the final vote on a man's entry. The initial interviewing and screening was still to be done by the warden and, where necessary, by a psychiatrist. The first selection meetings after this were anxious, nervy and somewhat frightening for all involved, particularly the potential new resident. Gradually, however, a system was evolved whereby each resident spoke a little about himself and the house before the applicant was asked to say anything. The applicant then explained why he wished to join the community and questions were asked of him, and he would then be taken to the kitchen for a cup of tea by a fellow-resident. A majority vote was next taken on his selection. Throughout the 18 months that this selection system has operated, only three men have been rejected. The house has not consciously raised its criteria of initial selection.

2 Discharge policy

During the first year the only definite rule was that a man would be asked to leave if he was known to have brought drink into the house. Each individual case was to be considered on its merits. The result was that some men were given two or three chances, while others were given seven or eight. No rules were laid down about such problems as violence, employment, gambling; no man was asked to leave for unsatisfactory conduct in areas other than drinking. Tension would develop between those who stayed very short periods or drank regularly, and those who seemed to want to make a determined effort to stay sober for relatively long periods.

During the second year, the whole problem of whether a man should be given a certain number of 'chances' or none at all was debated long and often. As one resident said, the house at one stage had become 'a convalescent home for drunks'. After about 18 months the men agreed at one house meeting that only 'one chance' should be given, but the residents knowing that they could drink once and return to the house, did just that. All of us became extremely confused as to what the house was really trying to achieve. Finally, towards the end of the second year, it was unanimously agreed by all the residents, and has been re-affirmed regularly ever since, that there was to be one rule of no drinking at all. As the figures for the third year in Table 20.1 show, this rule had undoubted benefits for the stability and sobriety of the residents in the house. But it was the resident group decision that was of cardinal importance. A staff-imposed rule of no drinking, which is only acquiesced in by the residents because they have no alternative, is very difficult to enforce, and is very likely to intensify staff–resident division.

In the third year it became necessary to consider whether there should be any limit to a man's length of stay. This arose because a small number of sober men seemed to be settling happily into the house. The residents' views on this issue were unmistakably clear: a fixed time limit produced anxiety and tension, and to avoid this situation a man should be allowed to decide for himself when he feels strong enough to leave. This was the policy that was adopted.

3 Group involvement

From the very beginning it had been intended that there should be a regular

127

weekly house meeting, at which all residents and the staff, including the visiting psychiatrist, should attend. It was to be run by the psychiatrist with a general discussion of house problems, and the residents' difficulties. In the first year these meetings generally met with an unenthusiastic response, a lack of interest and a desire to avoid them, if possible.

During the second year, we concentrated very much on making the house meeting a truly business meeting. One of the residents was elected chairman, and one as secretary, with the former being responsible for the general conduct of the meeting, while the latter produced minutes of each week's meeting. An agenda was prepared by the secretary and the warden, with all men being free to suggest items for it. This simple, but useful, structure gave the group a task at which it could now work. We moved clearly away from any notion of a sophisticated group therapy session, although this is not to say that in the discussion of items such as the redecoration of the dining room strong feelings and personality conflict were not shown. Gradually, however, it came to be seen that the ability of the house as a whole to make decisions, however small, was an important part of sobriety and that, once having made the decisions, we should keep to them.

The value of the residents' corporate involvement in the house was particularly illustrated in the second year when the group became interested in developing an Alcoholics Anonymous group in the house. This was to be run by the men and, as far as the residents were concerned, attendance at this meeting was voluntary, although for over a year the majority of the men attended. There can be little doubt that the influence of the AA group on the life of the house was healthy and beneficial. It undoubtedly gave a positive tone to general discussions in the house, which in the past had tended to be exclusively nostalgia for bomb-site escapades.

4 The warden's role

In the first year, all the staff were virtually in positions of total responsibility which made them paternalistic and authoritarian, however hard they tried to be otherwise. They took all the decisions, large or small. While such a staff role might be appropriate for some men, it was felt that to continue with such a role would prevent progress. Therefore, during the second year the residents, through the house meetings, were encouraged to become more involved, more willing to take decisions and accept responsibilities, and more committed to the idea of sobriety, enabling the warden in particular to abandon his earlier role. There was in particular a general retreat by the staff from small decision-making. The men answered the door and the telephone, had their own door keys, organised the weekly laundry, took messages,

128

entertained guests, did some of the shopping, and when staff were away, collected the rent. On several occasions they did the most difficult job of all – dealing with the drunken man. The warden ceased to be a round-the-clock supervisor and supporter. He became, in a sense, the social architect of the house. Such was the progress in this particular area that at the beginning of the third year, we were able to entirely abandon the idea of resident staff. The first year had begun with one house and three resident staff. The third year had begun with two houses and only one non-resident social worker.

5 The psychiatrist's role

As already indicated, two main functions of the psychiatrist were initially to give a thorough psychiatric assessment of any potential resident and to be the leader of the weekly house meeting. But as staff experience increased, the involvement of the psychiatrist in selection decreased. Outside the house meeting, the psychiatrist would see men individually where necessary. He also held a weekly staff discussion group at which the underlying dynamics of the house were discussed. Towards the end of the third year, the psychiatrist felt able to withdraw from the house meeting and merely held a weekly staff discussion group which came to accept their increasing responsibility. The development of the psychiatrist's role at Rathcoole suggests that in practical terms there may be no real need for a continuing and onerous commitment from a psychiatrist.

6 The general practitioner's role

Initially, it was expected that the residents would make heavy demands on the general practitioner. All men were registered immediately with the doctor and given a full, physical examination. Tests included a blood count, X-ray of the chest, electrocardiogram and liver-function tests. A full medical and social history was also obtained by the doctor. Surprisingly enough, the doctor found that the majority of men were generally in a good state of health upon arrival.

It is interesting to note that although in the first year some men did take antabuse, there has been no request for this drug for over two years, nor has any other form of drug therapy been encouraged. As the house has stabilised and the men have started to stay longer (see Table 20.1) the general practitioner has come to have a more significant role. He has become the family doctor and the men have enjoyed their visits to him for the minor ailments that afflict us all. The doctor has become a vital part of the

129

therapeutic team, rather than just a general practitioner who signs the sick notes.

7 The committee's role

At the beginning the committee consisted of a group of professional people concerned with and involved in the problem of the alcoholic. They gave invaluable support and guidance to the staff during the first year, not only at the monthly committee meetings, but also as individuals during the intervening weeks. As the experience and confidence of the staff increased, together with the support and involvement of the residents, the role of the committee became less certain. It appeared that there were two quite distinct functions. The first of these was administrative, legal and financial; while the second was therapeutic. It was felt that in matters directly affecting the life of the house, the residents, too, should be represented on the management committee and, accordingly, two men were elected on to it. The committee then became divided into two sections – one the house committee which dealt with the immediate day-to-day running of the house; the other, the finance committee, which looked at the long-term problems, financial and administrative. At the same time as this was happening at Rathcoole, another rehabilitation centre for alcoholics in a nearby borough was evolving a similar committee structure, and so it was decided to amalgamate experimentally the two house committees.

8 Lynette Avenue

As already mentioned, during the second year we opened another house with a capacity for eight men. With the new beginning we introduced the elements that we were finding useful and valuable at Rathcoole, i.e., selection by the residents, regular house meetings, non-resident staff and a rule of no drinking. We 'seeded' the house with two alcoholics who had been sober for a considerable period of time and who stayed for the first two months. This gave the necessary initial stability and meant that the first few residents arriving had some idea as to the real nature of sobriety and the ethos of the house they were joining. This policy proved successful and we were able, within a year, to have this house running as equally constructively and helpfully as Rathcoole at the end of three years. 'Lynette Avenue' was therefore a useful and vital addition to the whole experiment in that it showed that another house could be set up quickly and effectively, utilising the lessons of the first house. Development of Lynette Avenue was particularly encouraging in that no increase in staff was required, and that one social

130

worker was able to manage both this house and Rathcoole.

9 Staffing

It has already been made clear that Rathcoole began with a very high staff ration and that, gradually, this has been reduced, not because of financial necessity, but for therapeutic reasons. It is doubtful if the house could have begun with any fewer staff than it had and it is only the trials and tribulations of the staff in the first year or so that has made some of the subsequent development possible. Staff stability has been an important factor in Rathcoole's development as, clearly, it is difficult to establish growth with a succession of wardens. The first warden remained in post throughout the first three years, and the one assistant warden stayed for the 18 months that was required. The house also had the benefit of a succession of Community Service Volunteers who each gave about four or five months' service. The youth, enthusiasm and energy of the latter was particularly valuable, and it is in some ways a tribute to them that as the residents became more independent and responsible, the role of the Community Service Volunteer was increasingly an inappropiate one.

It is worth noting that if a small number of staff is justified as far as the effectiveness of the help being provided is concerned, it is also, of course, financially a great saving. During the first two years at Rathcoole, for example, the average cost per week, per man was usually between £16 and £18. During the third year, the weekly cost was about £11 to £12. The figures speak for themselves. However, financial benefits are, of course, not the only ones to consider. There are other implications that follow from having only one social-work staff member.

The most important of these is that there is a tendency for increasing responsibility to be thrown on to the domestic staff. At Rathcoole, for example, towards the end of the second year, a system had evolved whereby there was a non-resident housekeeper responsible for the cooking and the cleaning. She had limited contact with the residents and generally was well supported by the other staff. When, however, there was only one social worker for two houses, and he was non-resident, there was clearly an increasing responsibility thrown upon the housekeeper. She now had far more contact with the men.

The residents at Lynette Avenue, however, developed quite a different tradition as far as domestic staff were concerned. The house, itself, was physically very much smaller, although accommodating only two fewer men than at Rathcoole, which meant that the residents, themselves, felt able to take upon the responsibility for keeping the house clean. Further, as there

131

were no visitors, telephone calls or office work to be done there during the day, there was no real need for a full-time housekeeper, which meant that a part-time cook was a possibility.

10   Length of stay

Table 20.1 shows the breakdown during each year of the essential features of residency. It should be remembered that for the whole of the first year and for a considerable part of the second year, while a man might have been in residence with us for three, six or even 12 months, it is fairly certain that during this period, he would have had at least one, if not more relapses; whereas in the third year, in particular, the periods of residence reflect actual periods of sobriety. This is an important factor in interpreting the figures.

Table 20.1
Length of stay*

	1st Year	2nd Year	3rd Year
No. of admissions during year	35	45	18
Average bed occupancy	6.8	6.7	7.3
Average period of residence (weeks)	11	10	16
No. of men staying for:			
1 – 29 days	13	24	7
1 – 3 months	13	13	4
4 – 6 months	4	4	1
7 – 11 months	3	1	2
12 months+	2	3	4

* These figures apply to Rathcoole House only.

11   Occupancy rate

The level of occupancy within the house is a problem which can cause considerable concern to staff, residents and the financial supporters of the project. It is not often realised that a constant low-level of occupancy can demoralise residents as much as anyone. On one or two occasions during the first year, Rathcoole was reduced to two or three residents, and for a spell of a few days, only one resident. As Table 20.1 shows, the more stable a house becomes, the higher the level of occupancy it is able to maintain.

12   The future

(a)   *Are these houses for permanent residence?*

We may have to accept the fact that some men, if not many, will want to stay in our houses for several years if not for ever. There is a school of thought which says that men should come in for a given period of time and then be moved on, 'rehabilitated' completely. For the habitual drunkenness offender, this seems to be an unrealistic way of helping. If it is found from this experiment that men are most effectively helped by permanent residence in houses like Rathcoole, then this is something that should be accepted.

(b)   *The increased autonomy of the residents*

As suggested, it seems possible that the residents could in some circumstances be the almost complete managers of the house. This has been shown in other fields, notably by Merfyn Turner in his 'Second House'. There seems no reason to believe that former Skid Row alcoholics should not be capable of the same responsibility too.

(c)   *The future role of staff*

The staffing of any residential community, in this field or any other, has always been a major headache for the voluntary and statutory services. There would seem to be important lessons therefore, to be learnt from the third year of the Rathcoole experiment, when two houses were able to operate with one non-resident staff social worker. It ought to be possible in the future for several houses to operate possibly with one overall staff supervisor, and one or two assistants. There is no reason why one of these assistants should not, in fact, be someone who is being trained to run a similar house in another area. There is also no reason why the assistants should not be ex-residents of the houses themselves.

(d)   *The Rathcoole community extension scheme (alcoholics recovery project)* [1]

A successful application was made to the City Parochial Foundation in 1969 to obtain a grant for a three-year project which would seek to establish a comprehensive and co-ordinated system of help for the vagrant alcoholic. This will involve, for example, a co-ordinating centre for both the resources and the alcoholic in a given area of London. An attempt was urgently needed to assess the resources in one borough of London to see how far they met the needs of the homeless alcoholics in that area. It may be that a more efficient

133

and co-ordinated use of existing services could do a lot more to help the problem, whereas the temptation has always been to set up more and more new facilities, which in turn remain isolated from the other resources. In some areas of London there are 30 or 40 agencies – statutory and voluntary – any number of which might at any one time be dealing with one individual vagrant alcoholic. Further, it hopes to try to 'reach out' to the vagrant alcoholic, taking the help to him, rather than waiting for him to come to us.

(e) Prevention

From time to time we wonder whether enough preventive work is done. As it is estimated that only about three to five per cent of the alcoholics in this country are on Skid Row, it is reasonable to assume that there are factors other than just the alcoholism which have brought the man to that position. In this respect, the plight of the young Irishman coming to England deserves special mention and may give the clue to some areas of prevention that could be tackled. Not infrequently, the young, healthy Irishman coming to England can make a valuable contribution to the labour force. He has no roots, he is able to go from job to job and provide the hard backbone labour force for hydro-electric schemes in Scotland, London Underground projects, motorway building, and so on. When the particular job is over the man is paid off, has large sums of money but has no-one particularly with whom he can spend it, nor anywhere where he can rest and make good use of it. Possibly, for men like this, the community should think of setting up houses which can receive and help men to adjust to the kind of society which they probably find strange after a more rural, less hectic way of life in Ireland. These surely are the men for whom everything should be done to settle them into homely lodgings or special community houses. This is an example of an area to be looked at in preventive work. Certainly, in listening carefully to the personal accounts of the lives of Skid Row alcoholics, it is in areas like this that one feels that prevention could begin, rather than in the more confusing and uncertain area of warning young people against the evils of drink.

(f) The wider relevance of Rathcoole

It is generally agreed amongst observers and workers, both in and out of the prison service, that the vast majority of men in prison at any one time need not be there. The 'drunks' are a very small but nonetheless clear part of this group. If it is possible to show that prisons could be freed of the stage army of drunks that go through them and that these men could be helped to become useful citizens in the community outside, then not only could the prisons be free to do more work with other men, but they might also be encouraged to develop projects that tackle problems outside the prison walls rather than within them. Possibly, when all of us are bewildered by the failure of prisons to bring about any significant reduction in the rate of recidivism, or when we are shocked by the increasing borstal failure rate, we should pause and ask the reasons from the man or the boy who is bewildering and shocking us. They may have the answer.

Notes

[1] Further information on these developments can be obtained from Timothy Cook, 7 Klea Avenue, London, SW4.

21 Coping behaviour used by wives of alcoholics: a preliminary investigation*

JIM ORFORD and SALLY GUTHRIE

Summary

A standard 79-item multiple choice questionnaire was prepared as a means of eliciting information from wives of alcoholics concerning their own methods of coping with their husbands' alcoholism. The questionnaire was administered to 80 wives, items were intercorrelated and the resulting matrix subjected to a principal components analysis in an attempt to identify styles of reported coping behaviour. Rotation to oblique simple structure, using the Promax method, was performed and interpretation was attempted of the first five factors extracted which accounted for 27 per cent of the total variance. Inspection of item loadings suggested that all five factors could be meaningfully interpreted. Factor scores were calculated for all wives in the sample and these scores related to age and social class. Suggestions concerning the ways in which the validity of these factors might be established were discussed.

Introduction

The present paper is a report of a preliminary investigation into the ways in which wives of male alcoholics react to the consequences of alcoholism. A number of authors, such as Jackson (1954), Lemert (1960) and Bailey et al. (1962), have written about the adjustment made by the families of alcoholics but in none of these contributions has an attempt been made systematically to study individual differences in the behaviour of wives.

The purpose of the present investigation was (1) to develop a technique for eliciting information about the ways in which wives have coped or tried to cope with their husbands' drinking and its consequences, and (2) to find out whether, amongst the many behaviours to which wives resort, any broad styles of coping behaviour could be identified.

---

* A slightly abridged version of a previously unpublished paper of the same title, read at the 28th International Congress on Alcohol and Alcoholism, Washington DC, September 1968.

Method

Items of behaviour which were recognised by wives as ways in which they had behaved as a result of, or in an attempt to control, their husbands' drinking were collected by talking about the subject with individual wives whose husbands were under hospital treatment for alcoholism and with groups of wives who were attending meetings of Al-Anon in the London area. A list of 79 items was collected in this way, each of which had been mentioned by at least one wife to whom we spoke, and a 79-item questionnaire was prepared. Each item required the respondent to say whether she had ever behaved in the way described by the item and in each case one of four possible replies was required: yes often, yes sometimes, yes once or twice, or no.

The questionnaire was then administered to a further sample of 80 wives of alcoholics, names and addresses of whom were obtained from a variety of different sources; 71 per cent of the sample were married, 13 per cent enforced separation (husband in prison or hospital); 17 per cent separated or divorced; 13 per cent were in social class I; 21 per cent II; 34 per cent III; 10 per cent IV; 21 per cent V (Registrar General's Classification). The ages of the wives in the sample ranged from 20 years to 65 years with a mean of 42 years. In 55 cases the questionnaire was completed at the time of a visit by one of the authors (SG) to the wife's own home. In the remaining 25 cases the questionnaire was sent and returned by post.

Results

A score of three was given for a 'yes often' response, two for 'yes sometimes', one for 'yes once or twice' and naught for 'no'. Product moment correlations were computed between scores for every possible pair of items, thus yielding a 79 times 79 correlation matrix. Of the correlations in this matrix one in every 5.7 was significant ($p < 0.05$). It was concluded that a sufficient number of significant correlations existed in this matrix to justify principal components analysis of the matrix in an attempt to identify possible styles of coping behaviour used by the wives in this sample. The principal components produced by such an analysis were rotated to oblique simple structure using the Promax method (Hendrickson and White, 1964).

The first five rotated 'factors' accounted for 27 per cent of the total variance and these are summarised in Tables 21.1 to 21.5 where the ten items with the highest loadings on each factor are given with their loadings. [1] Each of these five factors appears to lend itself easily to subjective interpretation and consequently was given the label ('attack', 'withdrawal

137

within marriage', etc.) which is shown in the table. However, factor interpretation is notoriously a subjective and hazardous occupation and caution should be exercised in summarising a factor by such an arbitrarily assigned label. Whenever possible reference should be made, not to the label but to the factor loadings of individual items.

Five factor scores were calculated for each of the 80 wives in our sample. These scores were computed by giving each of the ten items with the highest loadings on the factor a weight of one and scoring each of these items 3, 2, 1 or 0 as before. [2] The range of possible scores on each factor was therefore 30.

The relationship between factor scores and social class and age in our sample was investigated by dichotomising the sample into those scoring above and below the median on each factor and splitting the sample into three social class groups (classes I and II together, class III, and classes IV and V together) and into three age groups (those in their 20s and 30s together, those in their 40s and those in their 50s and 60s together). The value of chi square was calculated for each comparison of factor score and social class or age. The results are summarised in Table 21.6 where it can be seen that there was a significant tendency for social classes IV and V to score highly on factor 1, for social classes I and II to score highly on factor 4 and for the under 40s to score highly on factor 5. A similar investigation of the relationship between factor scores and marital status at the time of completing the questionnaire was not possible as the numbers in categories other than 'married and living with spouse' were not sufficient. The nature of the items loading most highly on factor 1 would suggest the likelihood of a relationship between scores on this factor and marital status but it seems that high scores on this factor cannot be entirely explained by the presence in our sample of some women who were separated or divorced from their husbands as of the ten women obtaining the highest scores on this factor five were currently living with their husbands and a further three were only temporarily separated due to their husband's hospitalisation or prison sentence.

Discussion

Evidence of styles of coping behaviour

A major purpose of this investigation was the identification of styles of coping behaviour used by wives of alcoholics. By a style of behaviour we had in mind persistent use of a number of behaviours having elements in common. For a certain item of behaviour to be considered part of a person's style it should be characteristic of that person's behaviour and it should have something in

138

common with other items of behaviour used by that person. The results of this preliminary investigation could probably be used either to support or to refute the notion that such styles exist.

On the one hand the five factors extracted together accounted for only 27 per cent of the variance; over 70 per cent of the total variance is therefore not explained by these five factors. One might conclude that if these factors represent styles of coping behaviour then they are not very broad styles; perhaps a wife's reaction to her husband's alcoholism is too specific, too individualised, for us to be able to categorise her as being a wife who responds with a particular style.

On the other hand the items loading most highly on these five factors are such that possible interpretations of the styles of behaviour which may be represented by the factors are easily made. This being so these factors should not be dismissed as being of no importance merely because they account for a small proportion of the total variance. The apparent size of the factor is determined not only by its real importance but also by the number and nature of other variables involved in the analysis. It may be that by attempting to construct a comprehensive item pool on the basis of pilot work, we included a number of items of little significance. The 27 per cent of the variance which it has been possible to account for may turn out to be that part of the total variance with the greatest explanatory and predictive usefulness. The further possible explanation for part of the unexplained variance is that a degree of error variance has been introduced by the choice of a self-report method of investigation. Such a method, although the most expedient at this stage of the investigation, leaves most room for the introduction of error due to misrecall and misrepresentation. Systematic error variance may also be introduced due to the existence of various response sets, such as the sets to over-report, under-report, or to minimise the reporting of behaviour perceived by the respondent to be socially undesirable.

The correlates of coping behaviour

The usefulness of these factors as representing styles of coping behaviour will ultimately depend upon our ability to demonstrate their relationship to other concurrently measured variables and their ability to predict events which have not yet occurred. Lazarus (1966) has suggested that the behaviour a person uses to cope with a stress situation depends upon the degree to which the situation prevents their expectations being fulfilled, the relative appropriateness of the various possible means of coping with the situation, and the personality of the stressed individual. These suggestions serve to generate hypotheses concerning the relationships that we might expect

139

between scores on the five coping factors presented here and other variables. It might, therefore, be supposed that the behaviour used by the wife of an alcoholic will depend upon her beliefs about how a husband should be expected to behave, and the degree to which these expectations are currently being unfulfilled as a result of her husband's alcoholism. It may be that a greater degree of stress is required for a wife to score highly on factor 1 than is necessary for a wife to score highly on, for example, factor 3. Concerning the relative appropriateness of alternative means of coping, Jackson (1954) has pointed out that the wife of an alcoholic finds herself in a situation largely undefined by society and in which few standards of appropriate conduct exist. If this is indeed the case then it may be supposed that the situation leaves ample room for personality factors to influence the style of coping behaviour adopted. Personality correlates of coping behaviour are therefore to be confidently expected. Most importantly, the coping behaviour used by a wife may influence such future events as the outcome of her husband's drinking problem and the future stability of the marriage. A not unreasonable hypothesis might be that coping behaviour of the type contributing to factor 3 carries a better prognosis for the marriage and for her husband's drinking than does coping behaviour contributing to factor 2. These hypotheses and others concerning the correlates of coping behaviour used by wives of alcoholics are currently under investigation by the present authors in a prospective study of a hundred alcoholics and their wives who are attending a family clinic for alcoholism for the first time.

A start has been made in the present investigation to establish the correlates of coping behaviour by demonstrating the relationship in this sample between factor scores and age and social class. The degree to which these relationships are merely a function of this particular sample can only be determined by further investigation with fresh samples.

Notes

[1] It was thought possible that the results of the analysis might be distorted by the inclusion of items with extreme response distributions. A second analysis was therefore carried out with 17 items excluded, to each of which less than 20 per cent of our sample had given any other answer than 'no'. The first four factors produced by this second analysis appeared essentially similar to the factors 1, 2, 3 and 5 which are shown in the tables. Factor 4 did not appear from the second analysis.

[2] An alternative, and perhaps more accurate way of computing factor scores would have been to give all items weights proportional to the square of

140

their loading on a factor. However, in view of the preliminary nature of this investigation and the smallness of the sample and hence the possible unreliability of the factor loadings obtained, it was thought safest to adopt the system of computing factor scores which is described.

Table 21.1

Factor 1 ('attack')

Have you been legally separated?	+.63
Have you consulted a solicitor or advice bureau about getting a legal separation?	+.62
Did you try and stop him drinking too much by pretending to be drunk yourself?	+.61
Did you lock him out of the house?	+.60
When your husband gets drunk did you ever refuse to share a bed with him?	+.58
Have you ever left home, even for one day?	+.57
Did you refuse to sleep with him?	+.57
Did you pretend to everyone that all is well?	+.54
Did you ever try to hurt him physically?	+.53
Did you tell him he must leave?	+.50

Table 21.2

Factor 2 ('withdrawal within marriage')

Did you have rows with him about the drinking itself?	+.65
Did you avoid him as much as possible?	+.64
When your husband gets drunk did you ever feel too angry yourself to do anything?	+.61
Did you have rows with him about problems related to his drinking?	+.59
When your husband gets drunk did you ever feel too hopeless to do anything?	+.58
When your husband gets drunk did you ever keep out of his way?	+.57
When he is sobering up, did you leave him to it?	+.57
When your husband gets drunk did you ever start a row with him about it?	+.54
When your husband gets drunk did you ever refuse to talk to him while he was in that frame of mind?	+.49
When your husband gets drunk did you ever leave him to it?	+.48

Table 21.3
Factor 3 ('protection')

When he brings drink home with him, did you ever seem not to mind, but take the first chance to get rid of it?	+.65
When your husband gets drunk did you ever make him comfortable, perhaps by giving him something to eat?	+.61
When he brings drink home with him, did you ever try and find where it is hidden?	+.56
When he brings drink home with him did you ever hide it?	+.55
When he is sobering up, did you give him a drink to help with the hangover?	+.53
When he brings drink home with him did you ever pour it away?	+.50
When your husband gets drunk did you ever get him to bed?	+.49
Have you asked his employer to step in?	+.49
Did you arrange special treats for him?	+.48
Did you try and stop him drinking too much by going out to fetch him home?	+.45

Table 21.4
Factor 4 ('acting out')

Did you try and stop him drinking too much by getting drunk yourself?	+.67
When he brings drink home with him, did you ever drink some of it yourself?	+.52
Did you try and make him jealous?	+.51
Did you try and stop him drinking too much by trying to keep up with him when he drinks?	+.50
Did you try and stop him drinking too much by making him feel small or ridiculous in public?	+.46
Did you go out by yourself or with others and pretend to be having a whale of a time?	+.46
Have you had contact with Al-Anon?	+.44
Have you ever tried to show him how you feel by threatening to kill yourself?	+.39
Have you threatened to contact anyone to try to stop him?	−.39
When he brings drink home with him did you ever make a firm rule that you do not allow drink in the house?	−.36

Table 21.5
Factor 5 ('safeguarding family interests')

Did you yourself go without to give him the money he asked for?	+.66
Did you keep the children out of his way as much as possible?	+.64
Did you hide valuables or household things so that he couldn't pawn or sell them?	+.64
Did you pay his debts or bills?	+.64
Have you consulted a solicitor or advice bureau about getting a legal separation?	+.56
Have you tried to make other special arrangements about money matters?	+.51
Did you tell him the children will lose their respect for him?	+.39
When your husband gets drunk did you ever start a row with him about it?	−.36
Did you try and stop him drinking too much by inviting friends or relatives in?	−.35
Did you go out to work or use your own income to keep the family going?	+.31

Table 21.6
The relationship of factor scores to age and social class
(the significance of chi square)

	Factor	Age	Social class	Groups with high factor scores
1	('Attack')	NS	0.05	Social classes IV&V
2	('Withdrawal within marriage')	NS	NS	—
3	('Protection')	NS	NS	—
4	('Acting out')	NS	0.01	Social classes I & II
5	('Safeguarding family interests')	0.05	NS	Under 40s

22   Alcoholics known or unknown to agencies: epidemiological studies in a London suburb*

GRIFFITH EDWARDS, ANN HAWKER, CELIA HENSMAN, JULIAN PETO and VALERIE WILLIAMSON

Summary

Two parallel epidemiological investigations into prevalence of abnormal drinking were conducted in the same London borough. The first enquired of a wide spectrum of 'reporting agencies' the number of cases coming to their notice over a 12 month period, while the second study involved house-to-house interviewing and elicitation of subjects' own report of troubles experienced with drinking during the previous 12 months. The reporting agency survey revealed a 'labelling' prevalence per 1,000 adults aged over 16 of 8.6 for men, 1.3 for women, and 4.7 overall. About half these cases were known to a medical agency. The sample survey gave a prevalence of 'problem drinking' per 1,000 adults aged 18 or over of 61.3 for men, 7.7 for women, and 31.3 overall. The likely ratio of 'needful cases' to cases in contact with an 'apposite agency' probably lies between 4:1 and 9:1. The relevance of these findings to the planning of society's response is discussed.

Introduction

We present here some findings from a 'reporting agency' survey of alcoholism, carried out in one London borough. Results will be interpreted in the light of a house-to-house sample survey which was conducted at the same time, and in part of that same area. The extent of overlap in case identification will be closely considered.

Methodology of the reporting agency survey

Geographical area of study

To qualify for inclusion in the survey's count the primary criterion was that the subject should have (or have had at some time during the study year) an

---

* Shortened version of a paper of the same title originally appearing in the *British Journal of Psychiatry,* vol. 123, 1973, pp. 169–83.

144

address which fell within the boundaries of the old borough of Camberwell. A second type of subject was however also separately counted – the person who came to the notice of a Camberwell reporting agency, but who was of 'no fixed abode'.

The study period

The subject had to be reported as having evidenced symptoms of problem drinking between the dates 1 April 1965 to 31 March 1966.

Criteria for case identification

The basic criterion here was that one (or more) of the chosen reporting agencies should have identified the person concerned as having a notable drinking problem – the count was therefore primarily an enumeration of *labelled* persons. The reporting agents were not necessarily themselves expected to use the word 'alcoholism', but they were usually by inference making that diagnosis, if by alcoholism is meant simply that, as a result of drinking, the individual had suffered more than transient or trivial impairment of physical or mental health, or of social adjustment. A proportion of cases were however accepted for which the evidence was only of some acute episode (e.g., drunkenness arrest), and these cases are in the subsequent analysis separately categorised as 'casual'. Enquiry ensured that cases were not included in the count if the labelling was based on flimsy or non-existent evidence.

Choice of reporting agency

The word 'agency' will here be taken to embrace all individuals, institutions and other information sources employed in the study. The majority of the reporting agencies were sited actually within the borough but where necessary agencies situated outside the borough boundaries were contacted if they were likely to have involvement with Camberwell's alcoholism problems: obviously in all such instances only Camberwell residents were accepted for the study's enumeration.

The agencies finally selected were in summary as follows, with the numbering corresponding to that employed in Table 22.1: (1) *Courts:* four relevant magistrates' courts, Inner London Sessions, and the Central Criminal Court. (2) *Newspapers:* three local weekly newspapers were abstracted. (3) *General hospital casualty departments:* notes abstracted at two large local casualty departments and at two outside the borough. (4) *Probation service:* at all courts mentioned in (1) above. (5) *Clergy:* 65 contacted, with 56 of seven different denominations co-operating. (6) *Employers:* 290 Camberwell employers with more than ten people on the pay-role, and 15 large employers (more than 100 staff) in the neighbouring area. (7) *Local government welfare agencies:* education authorities, children's departments, welfare departments, housing authorities, reception centre (Camberwell residents only). (8) *Local government non-medical health agencies:* mental welfare officers, health visitors, public health inspectors, district nurses. (9) *Voluntary welfare, non-specialised:* five university settlements, two Samaritan organisations, one old people's welfare agency, three family case-work agencies, three counselling centres, two children's agencies, one ex-service agency. (10) *Voluntary alcoholism agencies:* three counselling centres and two rehabilitation hostels, all but one of these five being outside the borough. (11) *Alcoholics Anonymous:* local group and local intelligence. (12) *General practitioners:* 99 practices contacted in Camberwell and closely neighbouring areas with 97 co-operating. (13) *Psychiatric hospitals and psychiatric departments:* detailed abstraction from three psychiatric hospitals and three psychiatric departments serving the area and enquiry at six other general psychiatric hospitals and four specialised alcoholism treatment units: enquiry at three further psychiatric departments of general hospitals in the neighbouring area. (14) *General hospitals:* detailed abstraction from four hospitals serving the area and enquiries at 11 further hospitals. (15) *Prison medical service:* detailed enquiry at two prisons situated outside the borough regarding Camberwell residents or vagrants arrested within the Camberwell area, and at a third such prison taking only first offenders. (16) *Coroners' records:* abstraction at two coroner's courts.

Eliciting the co-operation of reporting agencies

Time and effort was spent in talking through with reporting agencies the nature of the phenomena which they were being asked to observe. A variety of special schedules were designed either as inventories to be filled in by reporting agencies themselves or as interview schedules to be used by research workers when interviewing agencies. Each research worker then took responsibility for fostering a personal relationship with a certain group of agencies and for maintaining contact with those agencies throughout the study year. The actual names and addresses of all cases were requested, so that there would be no duplication of case count. Guarantee was given of absolute confidentiality.

Treatment of data

The following items were those taken for statistical analysis: (i) demographic characteristics: resident/vagrant, sex, age; (ii) agency or agencies reporting the case.

To summarise the type of contact between the drinker and the labelling agency, it is useful to group these agencies, and the following terms will be used (numbering again as in Table 22.1): (17) *'Casually' reported:* reported by courts, press, or by hospital casualty departments. (18) *'Socially' reported:* by employers, clergymen and all voluntary or statutory social agencies other than those specialised in the care of the alcoholic. (19) *'Conversantly' reported:* report by general practitioners; psychiatric and general hospitals (other than casualty departments); by Alcoholics Anonymous or by social work agencies specialising in the care of the alcoholic. (20) *'Medically' reported:* report by general practitioners, by psychiatric or general hospitals, and by casualty departments. Thus group (20) overlaps (19). The intended value of the groupings is simply that they may roughly convey and summarise the type of contact between the drinker and the responding society.

Results of the reporting agency study

The knowledge possessed by different agencies

Table 22.1 shows the number and percentage of cases reported by each agency, and then (column two), by each agency uniquely – in the latter instance the count is of cases known to that agency but to none other. In the lower part of the table (items 17–20) data are given in terms of the summary categories as already defined; here the first column provides a count of total cases known between all the agencies in the relevant category but with any duplication of counting by the category's several agencies excluded, while the 'unique' column gives the sum of cases known to one or more agencies of that particular category but unknown to agencies in any of the other categories.

1 *'Casual' report* (item 17 of Table 22.1): this source was of major importance as regards the vagrants, of some importance for resident men and of little moment for resident women.

2 *'Social' report* (item 18): employers, clergy and social work agencies unspecialised in alcoholism, had little contact with the vagrant (10 per cent and unique < 1 per cent), but quite considerable contact (and unique contact) with residents – 28 per cent of resident women had unique contact with these agencies.

3 *'Conversant' report* (item 19): 41 per cent of vagrants, 42 per cent of resident men and 61 per cent of women were known to a conversant source.

4 *'Medical' report* (item 20): 37 per cent of vagrants, 48 per cent of resident men and 60 per cent of resident women were known to a medical agency.

With resident men, the contribution to the denominator (527) made by the 174 men known only to courts, press or casualty departments should be noted. If these had been excluded, the percentages apparently known to the remaining agencies would have been increased, e.g., the psychiatric services would report (not uniquely) on 40 per cent of cases and the general practitioners on 21 per cent.

Prevalence

It should again be stressed that these results here are presented not as an approximation to the true prevalence of abnormal drinking, but as prevalence of labelling – the relationship which may exist between true prevalence and labelling prevalence will be considered later. Excluding vagrants, overall rate for men (8.6 per 1,000 aged 16 or over), is between six and seven times that for women (1.3). For the total adult population the overall prevalence rate (4.7) is approximately double that which comes from combined medical agencies alone.

Methodology of the house-to-house sample survey

The methodology of this survey has been fully described in chapter 2. The sample survey population was entirely within the study area of the reporting agency survey. Of 1,039 subjects aged 18 or over in the drawn sample 928 were successfully interviewed, a success rate of 89 per cent. The male sub-sample interviewed totalled 408 and the female 520. Using a structured form of questioning, enquiry was made into each subject's possible experience during the previous 12 months of 25 drink-related symptoms (see Table 2.4). A score of five such symptoms arbitrarily defined a 'problem drinker'.

Results of the sample survey

The sample survey identified 25 out of 408 men and four out of 520 women as having experienced five or more untoward consequences of drinking during the previous 12 months, and as thus qualifying for the arbitrary label of 'problem drinker'. Expressed in terms of prevalence per thousand adults aged 18 or over, the problem drinking rates in this sample are thus 61.3 for males, and 7.7 for females and 31.3 overall.

Results overlap

1 *Sample survey: occurrences suggesting agency contact.* From the statements by the interviewed male problem drinkers themselves, the

148

expectation might have been that at least seven (28 per cent) would have been detected in the reporting agency survey if that approach had been entirely efficient. Among the women problem drinkers, one admitted contact with some of these reporting agencies during the previous 12 months.

2 *Overlap between reporting agency and sample surveys case detection.* Only three out of 25 problem drinkers identified in the sample survey were also identified by the reporting agency survey. Of the 22 cases that went undetected, five are perhaps instances in which research workers failed to gain information from agencies which seem to have had information to give. In the remaining 18 cases there was no admitted evidence of agency contact.

Putting this in percentage terms, out of 25 male problem drinkers identified in the sample survey, 12 per cent (three) were also picked up in the reporting agency survey while 88 per cent (22) escaped double identification – that 12 per cent (three) might theoretically have been brought up to 32 per cent (eight) if the reporting had been more efficient. It is perhaps particularly remarkable that only 8 per cent (two) of these problem drinkers were reported by psychiatric hospitals (no evidence of inefficient reporting), while not even one of these 25 problem drinkers was identified by the GPs who co-operated in the reporting survey; (20 per cent (five) of subjects themselves stated however that they had received medical advice to cut down on drinking). It must be emphasised that the drinking problems being experienced by the troubled males who had no admitted medical contact during the previous year were in some instances gross and in 44 per cent (11 cases) there was evidence of well established or prodromal alcohol dependence as judged by self-report of morning shakes and morning drinking. The numbers involved in these various calculations are of course small, and statements in terms of percentage must be interpreted very guardedly. Of the four women identified as problem drinkers in the sample survey, none was picked up by the reporting agency enquiry.

Turning then to the converse situation, no man and one woman contacted in the household survey was identified by the reporting agencies without being detected by direct interviewing.

Discussion

Limitations of the study

The coincidental sample survey suggests that, for a number of reasons, a proportion of cases of which agencies are indeed aware are not being reported to the research worker. This is an important proviso when inference is being drawn from the seeming disparity between reporting agency and sample

149

surveys. It must also be remembered that despite the research design being such as intensively to cover a wide spectrum of agencies within the borough together with relevant agencies around its borders and further afield, in an arbitrarily demarcated area of a big city no such coverage is likely to be 100 per cent complete. A pilot household study in a neighbouring borough revealed that the attempt to locate people living in houses which were in multiple occupancy was excessively time-consuming. It seems possible that excluding that type of property may lead to some under-estimate of problem drinking prevalence, but this remains speculative. There is however no very strong case for supposing that the nature of the information which comes from the comparison of the two survey approaches is for this reason vitiated – the chosen sample showed a class and sex structure which was close to that of the borough as a whole. Extrapolation from work conducted in one borough and at one time to the national scene must of course be cautious.

Comparison with previous prevalence estimates

The Jellinek formula

The Jellinek formula gives an estimate of alcoholism prevalence which is based on cirrhosis death rate corrected by certain other factors. Applied to England and Wales, the Jellinek formula 20 years ago gave a prevalence of 11 alcoholics per 1,000 aged over 15 (WHO, 1951). Of that total, a quarter were believed to be 'alcoholics with complications' (i.e., with cirrhosis). It was stated that the factor by which the 'with complications' rate had been multiplied so as to arrive at the overall rate was something of a guess.

From the present reporting agency survey, the overall prevalence rate per 1,000 adults aged 16 and over is 4.7. The disparity with the Jellinek formula is evident, especially as some of the cases which are counted in the survey would not necessarily qualify for inclusion by the formula's criteria. When, additionally, the sample survey's prevalence estimate of 31.3 per 1,000 is then taken into the reckoning, the matter seems to become even more confused. How are these apparent contradictions to be resolved?

The reporting agency estimate can perhaps here be rather simply put out of the way by again making the point that this type of survey should not be seen as providing a poor estimate of alcoholism prevalence but a rather good estimate of a community's awareness of alcoholism prevalence: properly read, the reporting survey's result in no way contradicts the other two estimates for it is not seeking to measure the same phenomenon.

The seeming contradiction between the Jellinek and sample survey approach is then probably explained along somewhat the same lines: the two approaches are here actually not measuring the same pathologies. The definition of 'alcoholism' inherent in the Jellinek formula and of 'problem drinking' employed in the same survey are both equally arbitrary, will count some cases in common but will in other instances be mutually exclusive. The advantage of the survey approach is that it makes entirely public the nature of the cases which are being enumerated, while what in Jellinek's terms is meant by an 'alcoholic without complications' is not so explicit. It must of course additionally be noted that the Jellinek estimate for the United Kingdom is not up to date, and the prevalence in an urban area may well be above the national average.

Special mention must be made of the important report by Moss and Davies (1967) whose work provides, so far as we are aware, the only other example in this country of a survey employing more than one or two simultaneously reporting agencies.

The surveys made purposeful

Of what use is this research? In examining its possible practical implications the same headings will be employed as were used in a previous review (Edwards, 1973). Indebtedness to Morris's analysis of the uses of epidemiology must be apparent (Morris, 1957).

1   *Building awareness*

The data cannot be employed as basis for unthinking activism. Given, however, the most properly conservative interpretation of the data and all due insistence on methodological limitations, the message would seem to be that in a British urban community abnormal drinking sets a not inconsiderable problem, with the true prevalence likely to be underestimated by the community's agencies.

2   *The differentiation of syndromes*

To suppose that these researches are concerned with the enumeration of one simple pathological entity would be wrong and the evidence from the sample survey makes this clear. To define syndromes, cross sectional will have to be supplemented by longitudinal survey.

3   *Case directed responses*

(a)   *Cases at present known to agencies.* Turning to Table 22.1 there is clear indication that a proportion of cases at present known to agencies are only

151

notified by a 'casual' source. This can only be considered a satisfactory state of affairs if we regard those cases as 'not real alcoholics', as people who should not appropriately be put in touch with a treatment agency. Such evidence as we have would in fact suggest otherwise (Gath et al., 1968).

Table 22.1 showed that 19 per cent of male and 28 per cent of female residents were reported only by 'social' agencies. That these cases were not put in touch with more specialised help is matter for comment and without in any way implying that the care being offered was of necessity inadequate, the finding at least suggests the need to investigate the causes of this non-referral.

(b) *Residents: cases at present unknown to agencies.* An estimate of the ratio between total needful cases in the community and total cases at present known to an apposite agency must obviously depend on two sets of criteria each of which are rather arbitrary:

(i) Criteria which are to define 'the needful case in the community'. The five problem cutting point is arbitrary and it is likely that different readers would accept rather different proportions of those cases as constituting 'needful cases'. Rather, therefore, than stating the prevalence rate as 31.3 per 1,000 it might be given as say lying between 15 and 30 per 1,000.

(ii) Criteria for 'apposite agencies'. A generous assessment of the prevalence of cases in contact with apposite agencies might be arrived at by subtracting only the 'unique casual' prevalence from the total reporting agency prevalence, thus arriving at a prevalence of 3.3 per 1,000. The best provisional guess is therefore that the ratio of needful cases to cases known to apposite agencies lies between 4:1 and 9:1.

(c) *The special problem of the vagrant.* The reporting agency survey shows that over half the vagrants will be known only to the courts.

Prevention

The size of the problem revealed by these epidemiological studies suggest the inadequacy of a national response to alcoholism which gives so little urgency to prevention.

Planning for the future

In the light of present findings, to conceive the planning of the community's response to its drinking problem in terms of just a little more of what we are already doing may be insufficient. If these results were confirmed, it would be difficult to believe that sufficient psychiatric manpower could be found to meet the problem by setting up more specialised hospital services which operated simply within the present model.

A strategy which the epidemiological findings might seem to suggest as worth consideration would be the setting up of local agencies (situated either within or outside the hospital), which would have in essence the following twin responsibilities:

1   The integration, activation and support of those who are to help the alcoholic. The role of the specialist might be seen as that of someone who aided and abetted the setting up of a range of facilities to respond to a wide range of drinking syndromes. His job would be that of consultation, and rather than his seeking to persuade the community that only 'the expert' can help the drinker, his prime aim would on the contrary be to maximise the potential of existing statutory and voluntary agencies, and particularly of the community's own unstructured power to respond.

2   Responsibility for seeking out the person who is indeed in need of special help – those severely addicted drinkers who are already to be found in contact with inappropriate agencies (courts), as well as the hidden proportion at present in contact with no agency at all.

Such proposals leave of course most questions unanswered. We are still, for instance, very unsure as to the worth of any of our therapies, and the suggestion that more people should be brought into contact with helping agencies must be seen as also inviting a continuing and critical appraisal of the help which is put on offer.

The only way in which thinking on these matters will be carried forward is by research, and in particular by the carefully monitored community action experiment. The size of the problem would seem to merit intelligent investment in such explorations. Hopeful spending on remedies of uncertain worth supplied to a small minority of people in need, and this coupled with neglect of any concerted preventive policy – with a problem of dimension and complexity such responses as these have as little to offer as a nosegay against the plague.

Table 22.1
Number and percentage of cases reported by each source and by summary categories

Agency or category	Vagrants (n = 294)				Resident men (n = 527)				Resident women (n = 93)			
	Reported by this source		Reported by this source uniquely		Reported by this source		Reported by this source uniquely		Reported by this source		Reported by this source uniquely	
	n	%	n	%	n	%	n	%	n	%	n	%
1 Courts: 1–2 arrests	161	55	142	48	135	26	79	15	8	9	5	5
3+ arrests	31	11	13	4	23	4	3	1	2	2	—	—
All court cases	192	65	155	53	158	30	82	16	10	11	5	5
2 Press	5	2	5	1	59	11	13	3	3	3	—	—
3 Casualty departments	17	6	4	1	68	13	45	9	4	4	3	3
4 Probation service	12	4	—	—	56	11	19	4	4	4	2	2
5 Clergy	2	1	—	—	40	8	30	6	12	13	7	8
6 Employers	—	—	—	—	18	3	14	3	—	—	—	—
7 Statutory welfare	4	1	1	<1	34	7	3	2	7	8	2	2
8 Statutory non-medical health agencies	11	4	—	—	16	3	4	1	10	11	6	7
9 Voluntary welfare, non-specialised	3	1	—	—	17	3	10	2	10	11	8	9
10 Voluntary alcoholism agencies	22	8	12	4	32	6	10	2	2	2	1	1
11 Alcoholics Anonymous	2	1	1	<1	6	1	1	<1	—	—	—	—
12 General practitioners	4	1	2	1	73	14	41	8	22	24	11	12
13 Psychiatric hospitals	96	33	52	18	140	27	64	12	33	36	16	17
14 General hospitals, excluding casualty departs.	10	3	1	<1	27	5	8	2	9	10	4	4
15 Prison medical service	11	4	1	<1	6	1	1	<1	1	1	—	—
16 Coroners	—	—	—	—	5	1	3	1	2	2	1	1
17 'Casual' (1) to (3)	202	69	166	57	239	45	174	33	14	15	8	9
18 'Social' (4) to (9)	29	10	1	<1	160	30	98	19	40	43	26	28
19 'Conversant' (10) to (16)	119	41	79	27	222	42	169	32	57	61	43	46
20 'Medical' (3) or (12) to (14)	109	37	67	23	253	48	190	36	56	60	44	47

23   Appraisal

Chapter 19 indicates that only between one in four and one in nine of 'needful cases' are in contact with appropriate helping agencies. A critical appraisal of that report would of course show that several important methodological problems have only been imperfectly met, but that paper does at least point very directly to a whole line of research which needs further to be opened up. There has to date been quite inadequate exploration of 'what counts as a case' in the eyes of the community, and the community certainly has many different pairs of eyes. There has also been inadequate study of how such perceptions influence help-seeking by the person in need, and gate-keeping by the responding agencies. The practical consequences of such interactions are almost entirely without description: we do not know whether the GP's sensible advice is more or less effective than all the paraphernalia of the specialised clinic, whether or in what circumstances the court's blunt response may be as helpful as the social worker's interventions, let alone the nature of the ramifying and criss-crossing pathways which are the respective routes to GP, clinic, court or social worker. These neglected questions are at least as real and as important as the conventional treatment research focus on this or that hospital régime.

Treatment is just one sub-variety of social response to the alcoholic as he swings between sick and deviant role. The primary respondents and for all we know the most potent respondents comprise the alcoholic's immediate human environment, his family, friends, neighbours, workmates. The mechanisms of informal control have been little studied. Orford and Guthrie's investigation of the coping styles of alcoholic wives is interesting perhaps not only for its immediate content but also as an example of a research approach to the informal micro-control system. The research possibilities in this general area must be many.

The report on Alcoholics Anonymous is a first level descriptive study of a self-help organisation. Again, such organisations have to date been subjected to rather little research investigation. The processes by which they are established and the continued processes of their organisation, the processes of the individual's affiliation and disaffiliation, the self-help group as instrument of attitude change, would all seem to be matters which would repay study. It would be interesting to count the number of research papers on hospital treatment of alcoholism appearing in the last ten years as against the number of reports on AA, and then to put these figures against some estimate of the comparative alcoholic 'case loads' of the National Health Service and Alcoholics Anonymous. Research it seems, is not always where the action is.

The description by Cook of the early years of the Rathcoole experiment is an unusual example of a voluntary project in the alcoholism field itself providing a detailed account of its foundation and first experiences. There has since the nineteenth century been a strong tradition of voluntary involvement in alcoholism rehabilitation, and yet the extent to which all that compassionate, energetic and imaginative investment has been assessed remains to this day vestigial.

The common underlying message of these four papers must therefore be that even as the medical doctor has sometimes found it inconvenient to believe that patients have any existence outside the consulting room, so the alcoholism research worker whose concern has been treatment has been rather too focused on that small element in social response which is the formal and medical contribution. The research problems which have to be faced when the remit is properly broadened are no doubt enormous, but this is no excuse for a continued and almost exclusive research concern with hospital treatments and hospital patients. The research worker no less than the doctor needs to get out of his metaphorical white coat.

156

SMOKING STUDIES

24   Introduction

Research into cigarette smoking was a latecomer to the Unit's spectrum of concerns, and hence the relative under-representation in the present volume of this important aspect of dependence studies. The papers have been chosen so as to illustrate a range of possible research approaches which may today be brought to bear on the smoking problem. The first paper proposes a 'strategy for future emancipation', and provides a broad perspective on the needed social policies and by implication the needed researches. Next follows an account of a pilot treatment trial which investigates a technique for treatment of the individual patient. A very different approach is suggested by a report on the influence of price on cigarette consumption, with its obvious implication for the population-directed public health approach. The paper on passive smoking suggests that cigarette smoking is fairly of rather more than just aesthetic concern to the non-smokers in the room. The report on the relationship between nicotine content of cigarettes and tobacco consumption and carbon monoxide yield, shows that a public health approach based on design of a 'safer' cigarette may have quite a few catches in it which will have to be solved before that approach becomes a real feasibility.

25   Smoking in Britain: strategy for future emancipation*

M. A. H. RUSSELL

Summary

The health cost of smoking in Britain, the national response to the problem and the reasons for failure to control it more effectively are discussed. A future anti-smoking strategy should hinge on the two interacting key factors that maintain smoking, the dependence factor and the favourable social climate. Any tactic or measure that diminishes the effect of either of these factors should also diminish smoking. In the absence of an effective treatment applicable to large numbers of dependent smokers and with lack of fundamental knowledge of the nature of dependence, our ability to overcome the dependence factor is at present rather limited. But much could be done to intensify research in this area. On the other hand, the engineering of a change of social climate to one less favourably disposed towards smoking is quite feasible and potentially highly effective.

Introduction

Clear evidence of the danger of smoking to health was provided over 20 years ago (Doll and Hill, 1950). Since this time with the help of two reports by the Royal College of Physicians (1962 and 1971), the case against smoking has been consolidated. Yet smoking remains widespread in this country.

The health cost of smoking

Whether or not the smoking of cigarettes is harmful to health is no longer at issue. The emphasis has now shifted to assessing the extent of this damage. Part of the price Britain pays for smoking is as follows:

(i)   It has been claimed by the Chief Medical Officer that nearly 100,000 people in Britain die each year before their time as a result of smoking (Godber 1970a). If this estimate is correct, smoking kills almost as many

---

* Based on a shortened version of a paper of the same title which originally appeared in the *British Journal of Addiction,* Vol. 66, 1971, pp. 157–66.

British people each year as the total number of civilians killed by enemy action during the whole of the last war (106,927 Central Statistical Office, 1951; 60,595 O'Brien, 1955). A more modest but nevertheless alarmingly high estimate has been made by Professor Lowe (1970). Using the excess mortality figures of smokers in an American prospective study (Hammond, 1966) and applying them to the mortality data for England and Wales, he calculated that some 38,000 men (24,503 under 65) and 4,000 women (2,678 under 65) die prematurely each year as a result of smoking. This is over five times the death rate due to road accidents and more than eight times the suicide rate (7,368 and 5,056, respectively, in 1968; Central Statistical Office, 1969). Lowe's figures are very similar to those given in the Royal College of Physicians' second report, namely between 20,000 and 24,000 premature deaths a year in men aged 35 to 64 caused by cigarette smoking. These 'smoking deaths' are mainly due to lung cancer, chronic bronchitis and ischaemic heart disease. Smoking is probably responsible for nine out of ten lung cancer deaths, three out of four bronchitic deaths and one in four deaths due to heart attack. Continued smoking takes an average of four years off the life of a young man – seven years if he smokes over 40 a day (Lowe, 1970; Godber, 1970b).

(ii)   Apart from the death rate there is the increased morbidity due to smoking. It has been estimated that the number of working days lost annually through illness directly attributable to smoking is more than 20 times the number lost through industrial disputes (Godber, 1969). Added to the personal suffering and financial cost to industry is the enormous extra burden on the Health Service for both outpatient and inpatient care of those who are ill as a result of smoking. Ball (1970) has estimated that between 5,000 and 8,000 hospital beds are occupied each day by smokers who are in hospital with illnesses they would not have had if they had not smoked. He has furthermore pointed out that this almost equals the complement of beds of the 12 London teaching hospitals.

(iii)   It is not only that the smoker harms himself. Besides producing smaller babies, mothers who smoke almost double the chance of their pregnancies ending in abortion, stillbirth or neonatal death (C. S. Russell et al., 1966).

The national response to the smoking problem

Smoking is not only harmful to health, in Britain taxation ensures that it is also expensive. How is it that despite these disincentives smoking remains so widespread? This is largely due to an interplay of two main factors.

(i)   *The dependence factor:* the nature of cigarette smoking as a dependence disorder results in the sad fact that it is difficult for the individual to stop.

Thus while three out of four smokers wish to or have tried to stop in the past, less than one in four ever succeeds (Russell, 1971a).

(ii) *The favourable social climate:* government apathy, vested interests and extensive commercial advertising not only encourage denial and distortion of the true facts but also subtly propagate false facts. The result is that the prevailing social climate in this country is one of approval and tolerance of smoking. There are not many places where smoking is not freely permitted. Cigarettes are perhaps the most readily available of all commodities.

Attempts to deal with the situation have been made on a number of fronts: treatment of the individual smoker, large-scale health education programmes and social control.

1 *Treatment*

After the 1962 Royal College of Physicians' report some 30 anti-smoking clinics were opened by local authorities throughout Britain. With few exceptions they all closed within five years due to disheartening results and lack of government support. A low success rate is common to smoking treatment clinics in other countries. The general experience is that of those attending such a clinic some 30–40 per cent stop smoking by the end of the course of treatment but by follow-up at one year the success rate dwindles to a range of 12 to 28 per cent (Berglund, 1969; Schwartz, 1969; Russell, 1970). Bearing in mind that the natural discontinuance of smoking within the British population at large is about 18 per cent (Russell, 1971a) it seems that the achievements of these clinics are rather limited. The prevailing state of therapeutic doldrums is reflected in the fact that there are no more than three or four smoking treatment clinics currently active in the whole United Kingdom.

These disappointing results are partly due to the limitations of the treatment procedures but another reason is that it is usually the most difficult cases who seek treatment. They tend to be not only highly dependent, but are frequently neurotic, depressed or beset by social problems that make it impossible for them to apply the necessary sustained effort to the task of withdrawal. A high relapse rate is one of the features of the failure of treatment. There is little doubt that this problem would be reduced if the general social climate was changed to one less favourably disposed towards smoking.

2 *Anti-smoking propaganda*

Smoking is so widespread that health authorities have rightly been attracted to the potential efficacy of large-scale anti-smoking propaganda programmes. These have been aimed in two directions – the persuasion of established smokers to stop and the prevention of children from starting. So far these attempts have met with discouragingly limited success. Straightforward dissemination of information about the multiple hazards of smoking seldom has the desired effect whether pitched at schools, communities or the population at large. Preventive propaganda in schools using films, posters and talks by health officials have been largely ineffective (Jeffreys et al., 1967; Holland and Elliott, 1968). A £4,350 community campaign in Edinburgh produced some change in attitude but no reduction in smoking (Cartwright et al., 1960). At a national level there have been spasmodic radio and television programmes and periodic poster campaigns which were able to produce attitude change in some smokers (McKennell and Thomas, 1967). However, a co-ordinated anti-smoking effort of significant magnitude has not yet been attempted on a national scale in this country. £100,000 a year of government funds to persuade people not to smoke is unlikely to achieve much in the face of the £12 million spent annually by the tobacco companies on advertising (Media Expenditure Analysis, 1970).

Lack of sufficient funds to pay for adequate and persistent exposure of propaganda messages has not been the only deficiency in anti-smoking campaigns. They have also lacked sophistication. But lessons are being learnt. Behaviour scientists interested in smoking problems are taking note of the growing field of communication theory and in their work on smoking modification they are contributing to that theory. The bulk of this work is, however, going on in the USA. There is in Britain virtually no active research in this area though it is obviously of great relevance to the health education field.

It is no longer expected that simple communication of facts will invariably induce appropriate changes in attitude or that a shift of attitude will lead to a corresponding modification of behaviour. The effect of a communication depends on an interplay of variables involving the nature of the informant, the type of message and certain characteristics of the recipient. Two useful reviews of the subject have recently come from America (Leventhal, 1968; Higbee, 1969).

In their outstanding survey of smoking habits and attitudes of adults and adolescents in England and Wales, McKennell and Thomas (1967) have suggested guidelines for improving future anti-smoking campaigns. They found that over 90 per cent of smokers are already aware of the association of smoking with lung cancer but that many are defensive and deny the relevance of these risks to themselves. To attack these defences directly, they advise, would be too threatening and therefore counterproductive for the majority of defended smokers. They suggest that more emphasis should be placed on minor health ailments such as cough and breathlessness, which many smokers are already experiencing. More prominence should also be given to the 'expense theme'.

Another possible reason for the relative failure of anti-smoking campaigns is that they may have placed too much emphasis on the rational cognitive reasons for not smoking, while the dominating and often unconscious social and psychological motives that determine the onset of smoking have been largely overlooked. The lesson of commercial advertising should perhaps be heeded. Repeated association of smoking with maturity, success, toughness, attractiveness and sophistication, etc., appeals to both conscious and unconscious needs. A recent survey (Bynner, 1969) has shown that schoolboys are indeed partly motivated to smoke by the image of toughness, sexiness and precocity that smoking provides.

In summary, to be more successful future anti-smoking campaigns should employ some of the methods of commercial advertising. This would be expensive as it would involve frequent, persistent and widespread exposure of propaganda messages as well as sophisticated application of the principles of communication theory. It would also require continuous monitoring of public response to allow feed-back control and adjustment of both form and content of propaganda messages.

3   *Social control*

The favourable image and omnipresence of smokers and smoking is a major factor in the recruitment of young people into smoking, in deterring established smokers from trying to stop and in seducing recent ex-smokers back to smoking. We cannot as yet do anything to alter the pharmacological effect of nicotine; this leaves the engineering of a change of social climate as the only practical way of curbing smoking on a massive scale. Advocacy of such social engineering is most difficult on ethical grounds, for it involves direct legislative intervention in the form of control of sales and advertising, banning of smoking in public places, and use of discriminative taxation; it therefore trespasses on the rightly sensitive area of infringement of personal liberty. A number of different means of social control will be considered:

(a)   *Restriction of tobacco advertising.* If the government does not choose to pay the enormous sum that would be necessary to compete adequately with the tobacco companies, the alternative is to restrict or ban tobacco advertising. A start was made in August 1965 when a ban was imposed on the advertising of cigarettes on commercial television. The tobacco industry responded with a massive proliferation of gift coupon schemes and there is no evidence that this tentative step by the government achieved any diminution in smoking prevalence, tobacco consumption or even cigarette consumption

(Russell, 1971b). For worthwhile results to be achieved it may well be necessary to not only ban all forms of cigarette promotion but to accompany this with extensive anti-smoking propaganda of a commercial advertising type and scale.

(b) *The role of taxation.* Judicious tax increases with the specific purpose of curbing smoking would be likely to be highly effective though somewhat harsh (see chapter 28). Selective tax increases to favour safer ways of smoking are more feasible. That this can be successful is amply demonstrated by the recent swing to the use of filter-tipped cigarettes.

(c) *Other legislative measures.* Pressure is being brought to bear in parliament for Britain to follow the American example in having nicotine and tar content as well as warnings of health hazards printed on all cigarette packets. There is lobbying for other measures such as banning of smoking in certain public places and pressure for tighter control of sales outlets, for example, the banning of cigarette vending machines. This would help reduce children's access to cigarettes directly; it would also encourage tobacconists to pay more heed to the law that already forbids them from selling to children under 16 years. All these measures would collectively contribute to make the public more aware of the disadvantages of smoking and thereby help to undermine the favourable social climate. Surprisingly, a majority of the smoking public and virtually all non-smokers would find many of these measures acceptable (McKennell and Thomas, 1967).

Suggestions for future anti-smoking strategy

Whether we are concerned with treatment of the individual smoker, with mass persuasion of the smoking population to stop, or with prevention of young people starting, for greater success, we are always brought back to the interplay of the two key factors that maintain smoking, *the dependence factor* and *the favourable social climate.* It is on these factors that a future anti-smoking strategy should hinge. Any tactic or measure that can diminish the effect of either of these factors should also diminish smoking.

Of the two, the dependence factor is probably the most refractory owing to current lack of fundamental knowledge of the nature of dependence. Research in this area and into more effective treatment would be an important part of the wider strategy. About 50 per cent of smokers acknowledge the disadvantages of smoking and wish to stop (McKennell and Thomas, 1967). If an effective 'smoking cure' were developed, these dissonant smokers would no doubt come swarming to get it. By virtue of their numerical strength alone current smokers contribute to maintaining the social climate favourable to smoking. By substantially reducing the number of smokers a more effective treatment of smoking would, therefore, have the bonus effect of helping to change the social climate away from acceptance of smoking.

Some of the problems of communication have already been mentioned. A programme would need to be linked with social research including continuous evaluation and public reaction monitoring. Social research soundings would probably indicate that different sorts of message are required for people of different ages. Possible ancillary tactics might include restriction of cigarette sales outlets, banning of smoking in certain public places, warnings printed on cigarette packets, etc. But each of these measures would require careful consideration and testing of public acceptability before introduction, for the essence of good communication is to avoid backlash effects.

Just as successful treatment of large numbers of dependent smokers would contribute to changing the social climate, so would a change in social climate facilitate treatment. Once a change in social climate and the image of smoking was wrought, increasing numbers of mildly dependent smokers would stop and fewer young people would adopt the habit. The initial phase of such a programme would be the most difficult, with later stages tending to be facilitated by a snowball effect.

The role of doctors would be of tactical relevance; as exemplars they affect the image of smoking, as informants of high credibility it would help if they took every opportunity to advise and encourage their patients to stop smoking. The power of simple but firm advice against smoking, given by a doctor to his patients is such that it could well yield a success rate of up to 20 per cent (Russell, 1971c). If each of the 20,000 general practitioners in England were to persuade but one patient a week to stop smoking, the yield would be over 1,000,000 ex-smokers a year. To equal this it would require 10,000 anti-smoking clinics each having a 33 per cent success rate with 300 subjects a year.

Safer ways of smoking cigarettes, other than extreme moderation, should be regarded as no more than a temporary expediency for those who are unable to stop. Hopes for a 'safe cigarette' are to some extent misguided. It would solve only part of the problem in that a completely safe cigarette would have to be nicotine-free as well as carcinogen-free and most heavy smokers could as easily give up altogether as transfer to nicotine-free cigarettes. However, it would help if taxation favoured cigar and pipe smoking. It is possible that as social customs change and knowledge and experience is gained of both the dangers and the early stages of dependence, the large majority of us may, as is the case with alcohol, learn to limit our smoking to an occasional cigar or pipe. Indeed, many would consider this goal preferable to the abolition of all smoking.

Clearly the suggested strategy demands a co-ordinated, sustained and massive intervention on a national scale. It would require a multi-disciplinary organising committee closely backed by the government with generous financial and legislative support. Drastic and expensive though this may be, it would be a pity if the government allowed its reluctance to lose the £1,000 million-plus it annually derives from tobacco revenue to stand in the way of what is potentially the most important health measure that is likely to be open to us for the rest of this century.

26 Effect of electric aversion on cigarette smoking*

M. A. H. RUSSELL

Summary

Electric aversion was administered to 14 cigarette smokers. Six of the nine who completed the treatment were still abstinent at one year follow-up. The overall average of 21.5 cigarettes on the day before treatment dropped to an average of 1.4 cigarettes per day after the third aversion session, and most patients stopped smoking within five sessions. It is concluded that electric aversion is a powerful suppressor of cigarette smoking, but its use is limited to a small group of well-motivated smokers.

Assessment and selection of subjects

The fourteen subjects were chest clinic patients referred by their chest physicians for cigarette withdrawal. They had to show good motivation for treatment.

Methods

The shock box was a portable battery-driven multivibrator type. The strength of the shocks was determined by the subjects and was kept at a level which was unpleasant but not intolerable. Using a semantic differential attitude scale, attitudes to various concepts were measured at the initial assessment and again just before treatment; repeated measurements were made throughout the course of treatment and follow-up. All subjects were treated as outpatients. Sessions lasted about one hour. Treatment was continued until the urge to smoke was eliminated or rendered minimal (average 11 sessions over 27 days).

Aversion to smoking practice

After placement of electrodes on the left forearm an unpleasant but not

---

* Synopsis of a paper of the same title, which originally appeared in the *British Medical Journal,* Vol. 1, 1970, pp. 82–6.

intolerable shock intensity was selected. The subject was instructed to start smoking in his usual way. At any stage during the smoking act, from reaching for the packet, to lighting, to almost finishing the cigarette, a signal (pencil tap on desk) was given. This signal was followed in three out of four trials by a shock. The time interval between the signal and the shock was about half to one second. The subject was instructed to discard the cigarette immediately on receiving the signal. He was warned that any tardiness would incur a second shock. In practice this was rarely necessary, except in the first few trials. About 20 such smoking practice trials (involving 15 shocks) were performed each session.

Aversion to smoking fantasy

Each subject selected situations in which he found it was most difficult to do without a cigarette. He was asked to imagine himself smoking in such a situation, and to say 'now' when his fantasy reached the stage of lighting the cigarette. The moment he said 'now' he received the signal (pencil tap) followed in three out of four trials by the shock. Generally about ten trials (involving seven shocks) of aversion to a fantasy were completed each session.

Therapist's role

The therapist attempted to assume the role of a friendly but directive doctor and to convey confidence in the efficacy of the treatment and its ability to stop the subject smoking.

Results

Nine of the 14 subjects completed the course of aversion therapy, four dropped out, and one became so depressed that treatment was discontinued. Six subjects (43 per cent) were still off cigarettes at the follow-up period of one year. The success rate of those completing treatment was 67 per cent. All cases achieving one year of abstinence were checked by obtaining confirmation from a friend or member of the family.

Most subjects stopped smoking within five sessions but one required 14 sessions before stopping. In most cases there was an appreciable effect after the first session. All cases showed a striking shift of attitude to the concepts 'smoking' and 'cigarettes' (Figures 26.1 and 26.2) while attitude to non-smoking concepts such as 'tea' and 'mother' remained unaffected. Seventy-three per cent of the total attitude change had occurred by the end of the third session (mean of all subjects).

169

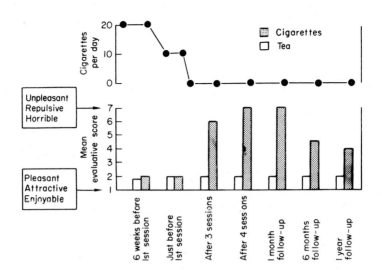

Fig. 26.1 Changes in smoking attitude and behaviour with aversion therapy in one subject.

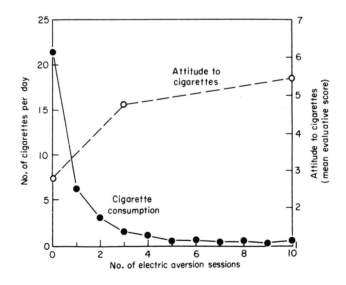

Fig. 26.2 Changes in cigarette consumption and attitude to cigarettes (expressed as 'mean evaluative score' derived from attitude scale) occurring during electric aversion therapy. Both curves derived from the mean of all subjects.

170

Anxiety was felt by most subjects, but there was great variation. Depression was the most troublesome side-effect of therapy and was experienced by eight of the subjects. It bore no relation to the outcome of treatment, but it was more frequent and severe in the women (occurring in three out of the four).

The results indicate that electric aversion suppressed cigarette smoking. This effect was probably due mainly to classical conditioning, but other influences (e.g., 'suggestion', relationship with therapist) were applied in an uncontrolled way. The use of aversion therapy is becoming widespread, yet it is still not known how or why it works in humans; whether by classical conditioning as in animals or by cognitive processes such as those involved in religious conversion, faith healing, and placebo response. Controlled trials are needed to identify and evaluate the effective elements in aversion therapy.

27 Changes in cigarette price and consumption by men in Britain, 1946–71: a preliminary analysis*

M. A. H. RUSSELL

Summary

Analysis of changes in the price of manufactured cigarettes and consumption by men in Britain over the 25 year period 1946–71 revealed a strong inverse linear relationship. An annual increase in 'basic' price of five per cent or more invariably depressed consumption. After correcting the price to 1963 values or by expressing it as a proportion of personal disposable income, negative correlations as high as 0.9 were found (P < 0.001). Regression coefficients showed that for every old penny change in the 'corrected' price of 20 cigarettes, consumption changed inversely by about 40 cigarettes per head per year; and that for every one per cent change in 'corrected' price, consumption changed inversely by about 0.6 per cent indicating that the demand for cigarettes is 'inelastic'. Both the 1962 and 1971 Royal College of Physicians' reports depressed cigarette consumption, the effects being respectively equivalent in potency to increases in 'corrected' price of 6.1 and 8.6 old pence for 20 cigarettes. Selective taxation to increase the price of cigarettes by about ten per cent a year is suggested as an essential ingredient for success in the control of cigarette smoking.

Introduction

The possibility of changing smoking behaviour by price manipulation has received relatively little attention. Since 1946, in addition to seven manufacturers' price increases, there have been nine increases in tobacco duty, some of them large. No systematic analysis has yet been published of the effect of these price changes on smoking behaviour and tobacco consumption. This paper presents a preliminary analysis of the effect of price on cigarette consumption.

---

* Condensed from an article published in the *British Journal of Preventive and Social Medicine*, Vol. 27, 1973, pp. 1–7.

Methods

The study was confined to analysing the relationship between price and consumption of manufactured cigarettes.

The consumption variable

Cigarette tobacco sales by weight is an unsatisfactory measure of the amount smoked. Less tobacco is used in filter-tipped cigarettes. Thus the trend towards filter-tipped cigarettes does of itself account for much of the decline in tobacco sales by weight, independent of any change in the amount smoked. The number of cigarettes sold is a more accurate measure of consumption in terms of the amount smoked.

During the period covered by this analysis the prevalence of smoking among women was rising. This was due to social forces that were probably largely independent of price. To obtain a purer measure of the influence of price, the analysis was confined to consumption by men. Per capita figures were used to correct for population changes over the years.

The final consumption variable selected was the *'consumption of manufactured cigarettes by men (aged 15 and over) in numbers of cigarettes per head per year'*. The figures were obtained from the Tobacco Research Council (Todd, 1972).

The basic price variable

Figures for changes over the years in retail price of 20 standard plain (non-tipped) cigarettes were obtained from Her Majesty's Customs and Excise (HM Customs and Excise Annual Reports, 1968–70) together with details of increases in tobacco duty and manufacturers' price (see Table 27.1). Similar figures have been published by the tobacco trade (Tobacco Trade Year Book and Diary, 1972).

The two sources tally except for the manufacturers' price increase in 1951 which is not included in the tobacco trade figures. Personal enquiry revealed that this was not included because some, but not all, manufacturers increased their prices at that time. It was not possible to obtain the proportion of the market held at the time by those manufacturers who did increase their prices. The tobacco trade source unfortunately refused to pursue the point so that it was not possible to set right the discrepancy. This 1951 price rise is also the only one for which the precise date is not known. It is known only that it occurred some time after June. For this analysis it was taken as 15 September.

With knowledge of the date and the amount of individual price rises it is possible to calculate the mean price of 20 standard plain cigarettes for each year. This price unit has been kept in old pence partly because the years analysed precede decimalisation but also because conversion to new decimal pence requires approximations which would have introduced needless loss of variance. For example, both two and three old pence each equal one new penny.

Instead of the mean price for each year of 20 standard plain cigarettes it would have been preferable to have used the mean price for each year of 20 cigarettes taking the mean from all types of manufactured cigarettes consumed during the year. This would have obviated loss of variance due to the shift towards smoking cheaper filter-tipped and small-sized cigarettes. For example, instead of smoking fewer cigarettes after a price rise, there is also a tendency to respond by switching to cheaper cigarettes without cutting down on the number smoked. Figures for this ideal basic price variable are unfortunately not yet available so that for this analysis the basic price variable used was the 'mean price for each year of 20 standard plain cigarettes in old pence'. This variable is referred to simply as the *'basic' price.*

Adjusted price variables

In an analysis involving price changes over time it is obviously essential to correct for the declining value of money. This was done by adjusting the 'basic' price to 1963 values, using the Index for Annual Internal Purchasing Power of £1 at 1963 value (Central Statistical Office, 1971a). This adjusted price variable is referred to as the *'corrected' price.*

Another approach used was to examine the effect of price relative to income by expressing the 'basic' price for each year as a percentage of annual per capita personal disposable income at current prices (Central Statistical Office, 1971b). This adjusted price variable is referred to as the *'price-income ratio'.*

The time span

The analysis covered the years 1946–71. The war years were excluded because the situation was so unusual and figures for the essential price adjustments are not available for the war period.

Results

Inspection of Table 27.1 shows that of the 25 years covered by the study annual cigarette consumption fell in ten and increased in 15. There were eight occasions when 'basic' price increased by five per cent or more. In all eight of

Table 27.1
Cigarette price and consumption changes for men in Britain 1946-71

Year	s.	d.	Date and Amount of Price Increase	Basic Price — Mean Price for Year (old pence, % annual rise)	Internal Purchasing Power of £1 at 1963 Value (% annual fall)	Annual per capita Personal Disposable Income at Current prices in £ (% annual rise)	Corrected Price — Mean Price for Year (old pence adjusted to 1963 value of £1, % annual change)	Price Income Ratio — Mean Price for Year (old pence as % of annual per capita personal disposable income, % annual change)	Consumption of Manufactured Cigarettes by Men (no. of cigarettes/head/year, % annual change)
1946	2	4		28.0	183.5	154 (7.14)	51.38	0.0758	4280
1947	3	4	D+12d 16 April (42.86%)	36.5 **(30.36)**	171.8 (6.4)	165 (7.14)	62.71 **(+22.05)**	0.0922 **(+21.61)**	3670 (−14.25)
1948	3	6	D+2d 7 April (5.00%)	41.5 **(13.70)**	159.5 (7.2)	172 (4.24)	66.19 **(+ 5.55)**	0.1005 **(+ 9.00)**	3520 (− 4.09)
1949	3	6		42.0 **(1.20)**	155.8 (2.3)	180 (4.65)	65.44 **(− 1.13)**	0.0972 **(− 3.28)**	3320 (− 2.84)
1950	3	6		42.0	151.5 (2.8)	188 (4.44)	63.63 (− 2.77)	0.0931 (− 4.22)	3370 (+ 1.51)
1951	3	7	M+1d After June* (2.38%)	42.3* (0.71)	138.9 (8.3)	204 (8.51)	58.75 (− 7.67)	0.0864 (− 7.20)	3610 (+ 7.12)
1952	3	7		43.0 (1.65)	131.1 (5.6)	218 (6.86)	56.37 (− 4.05)	0.0822 (− 4.86)	3640 (+ 0.83)
1953	3	7		43.0	128.9 (1.7)	233 (6.88)	55.43 (− 1.67)	0.0769 (− 6.45)	3690 (+ 1.37)
1954	3	7		43.0	126.6 (1.8)	245 (5.15)	54.44 (− 1.79)	0.0731 (− 4.94)	3740 (+ 1.36)
1955	3	8	M+1d 17 October (2.33%)	43.2 (0.47)	122.4 (3.3)	264 (7.76)	52.88 (− 2.87)	0.0682 (− 6.70)	3830 (+ 2.41)
1956	3	10	D+2d 18 April (4.55%)	45.4 **(5.09)**	117.2 (4.2)	282 (6.82)	53.21 **(+ 0.62)**	0.0671 **(− 1.61)**	3740 (− 2.35)
1957	3	11	M+1d 16 September (2.17%)	46.3 (1.98)	113.6 (3.1)	295 (4.61)	52.60 (− 1.15)	0.0654 (− 2.53)	3790 (+ 1.34)
1958	3	11		47.0 (1.51)	110.6 (2.6)	308 (4.41)	51.98 (− 1.18)	0.0636 (− 2.75)	3840 (+ 1.32)
1959	3	11		47.0	109.9 (0.6)	325 (5.52)	51.65 (− 0.63)	0.0603 (− 5.19)	3890 (+ 1.30)
1960	4	2	D+2d 5 April (4.26%); M+1d 12 June (2.04%)	48.5 (3.19)	108.8 (1.0)	347 (6.77)	52.77 (+ 2.17)	0.0582 (− 3.48)	4030 (+ 3.60)
1961	4	6	D+4d 26 July (8.00%)	51.3 **(5.77)**	105.7 (2.8)	369 (6.34)	54.23 **(+ 2.77)**	0.0579 **(− 0.52)**	4010 (− 0.50)
1962	4	6	(1st RCP Report) 7 March	54.0 **(5.26)**	101.8 (3.7)	383 (3.79)	54.97 **(+ 1.36)**	0.0587 **(+ 1.38)**	3750 (− 6.48)
1963	4	6		54.0	100.0 (1.8)	405 (5.74)	54.00 (− 1.76)	0.0556 (− 5.28)	3800 (+ 1.33)
1964	4	10	D+4d 15 April (7.41%); M+1d 9 August (1.72%)	57.2 **(5.93)**	96.8 (3.2)	432 (6.67)	55.37 **(+ 2.54)**	0.0552 **(− 0.72)**	3740 (− 1.58)
1965	4	11	D+6d 7 April (10.17%)	63.4 **(10.84)**	92.6 (4.3)	459 (6.25)	58.71 **(+ 6.03)**	0.0576 **(+ 4.35)**	3580 (− 4.28)
1966	5	5		65.0 (2.52)	89.2 (3.7)	484 (5.45)	57.98 (− 1.24)	0.0560 (− 2.78)	3640 (+ 1.68)
1967	5	5		65.0	87.0 (2.5)	502 (3.72)	56.55 (− 2.47)	0.0540 (− 3.57)	3740 (+ 2.75)
1968	5	7	D+2d 20 March (3.08%); M+1d 16 July (1.49%); D+5d 23 November (7.35%)	67.6 (4.00)	83.3 (4.3)	533 (6.18)	56.31 (− 0.42)	0.0528 (− 2.22)	3850 (+ 2.94)
1969	6	1		73.0 **(7.99)**	79.1 (5.0)	561 (5.25)	57.74 **(+ 2.54)**	0.0542 **(+ 2.65)**	3790 (− 1.56)
1970	6	2	M+1d 26 October (1.37%)	73.2 (0.27)	75.0 (5.2)	609 (8.56)	54.90 (− 4.92)	0.0501 (− 7.56)	3910 (+ 3.17)
1971	6	2	(2nd RCP Report) 5 January	74.0 **(1.09)**	69.6 (7.2)	674 (10.67)	51.50 **(− 6.19)**	0.0457 **(− 8.78)**	3710 (− 5.12)

* Calculated as 15 September

M = manufacturers' increase; D = increase in tobacco duty (see Note).

Note: For technical reasons associated with the structure of tobacco taxation, it is not possible to express the duty element on a packet of cigarettes in absolute terms. The figures of duty element shown in the Table are therefore approximate.

The % annual changes in bold type for three of the price variables represent those years in which consumption fell.

these years consumption fell. This association is unlikely to be fortuitous (P < 0.001, Fisher's exact test). Furthermore, for the two exceptional years in which consumption fell in the absence of a notable price rise there is an adequate explanation. In 1949 the effects were no doubt still being felt of the massive price increases of the two preceding years. The fall in consumption in 1971 was almost certainly due to the second report of the Royal College of Physicians.

The association is no less strong in the case of 'price–income ratio'. In each of the eight years that show a rise in the ratio or a fall of less than two per cent, there is a drop in consumption. Again 1949 and 1971 are the exceptions. For 'corrected' price the association with consumption is also strong on simple inspection, but 1960 appears here as a glaring exception that is not immediately explicable.

Figure 27.1 shows graphically the clear inverse relationship between consumption and 'corrected' price. The year of the second Royal College of Physicians' report, 1971, is the only one in which this mirror-image relationship is substantially disturbed. The relationship is quantified in Table 27.2 in the form of product-moment correlation co-efficients and regression co-efficients. It can be seen that a large amount of variance is accounted for by the enormous price and consumption change that occurred in 1947.

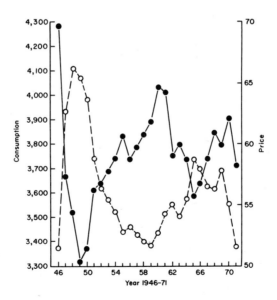

Fig. 27.1 Changes in 'corrected' price of cigarettes and consumption by men in Britain, 1946-71: cigarettes/adult man per year; O– –O mean price for year in old pence of 20 standard plain cigarettes corrected to 1963 values.

Excluding 1962 and 1971, the two years which witnessed the additional influence of the Royal College of Physicians' reports, changes in price account for some 80 per cent of the variation in consumption over the period studied.

The regression co-efficients (Table 27.2) indicate that for each one old penny change in the 'corrected' price of 20 cigarettes the consumption by men showed an opposite change of about 40 cigarettes per head per year; and that for every one per cent change in 'corrected' price, consumption changed inversely by about 0.6 per cent.

Table 27.2

Correlation and regression coefficients between cigarette consumption and price variables, 1946–71

	Consumption (no. of cigarettes/ head/year) v 'Corrected' Price† (old pence)	% Change in Consumption v % Change in 'Corrected' Price	% Change in Consumption v % Change in 'Price-Income Ratio'
Correlation Coefficients			
All years	−0.77**	−0.78**	−0.79**
Excluding 1947		−0.52*	−0.56*
Excluding 1962 and 1971	−0.80**	−0.92**	−0.91**
Excluding 1947, 1962 and 1971		−0.78**	−0.77**
Regression Coefficients			
All years	−35.59	−0.59	−0.53
Excluding 1947		−0.50	−0.44
Excluding 1962 and 1971	−38.23	−0.66	−0.58
Excluding 1947, 1962 and 1971		−0.65	−0.52

† For 20 standard plain cigarettes.   * $P<0.01$;   ** $P<0.001$.

The data comparing 'corrected' price with consumption and per cent change in 'corrected' price with per cent change in consumption for each year were plotted, together with the least squares regression lines, for the two sets of data (Figs. 27.2 and 27.3). The years which are out of alignment with the general trend are clearly evident. It seems that for 1949, 1962, 1971, and, to a lesser extent, 1956 some influence other than price was operating more strongly to depress consumption. It has already been suggested that the Royal College of Physicians' reports account for 1962 and 1971 and that 1949 could have been affected by the unduly large price increases of the preceding two years, but there is no obvious explanation for 1956. Likewise it is not clear why consumption was so high relative to price in 1960 and 1968.

Discussion

To have found an inverse relationship between the price of cigarettes and their consumption is not surprising. The interest of the analysis rests more in ascertaining the strength and nature of the relationship. The high negative correlation of 0.9 indicates that changes in price account for as much as 80 per cent of the variation in consumption by men over the 25 years between 1946 and 1971. The relationship appears to be linear rather than curvilinear, at least within the range of price change (−8 to +22 per cent annual change in 'corrected' price) that occurred during the period studied. This is rather unexpected and means that a price increase of 20 per cent does not depress consumption relatively more than an increase of one per cent. Moreover, the relationship seems to be the same whether the price change is upwards or downwards.

A persistent decline in the purchasing power of money and a rise in personal income over the years ensure that cigarettes become progressively cheaper in real terms unless the 'basic' price is increased in step with these economic trends. To exceed these trends requires a substantial increase in 'basic' price of five per cent or more. For the period studied, in all eight of the years that witnessed annual price rises of this order consumption was depressed (see Table 27.1). All eight of these large price increases were instigated by the Government. Manufacturers' increases, always less than three per cent, have been too small to depress consumption noticeably. On the four occasions that they were not contaminated by the effect of tobacco duty increases (1951, 1955, 1957, 1970) there was no evident fall in consumption.

Data on changes in smoking prevalence over the years are awaited before it is possible to assess how much the fall in consumption resulting from a price rise is due to established smokers reducing or stopping smoking and how much to a lowered recruitment to smoking.

Price and elasticity

As an index of the responsiveness of the consumption of a product to price changes, economists have developed the concept of 'elasticity' (Samuelson,

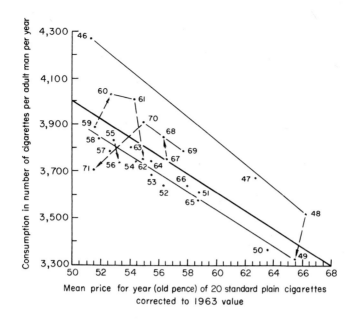

Fig. 27.2   Comparison of 'corrected' price and consumption of cigarettes by men, 1946-71.
Note: Each point on the graph represents one year. The bold line is the least squares regression line for consumption on price, excluding the years 1962 and 1971 (r = −0.80, P<0.001). Fine solid lines indicate the slope between consecutive years which approximately parallel the regression line. Arrowed broken lines show the years which aberrate from the general trend.

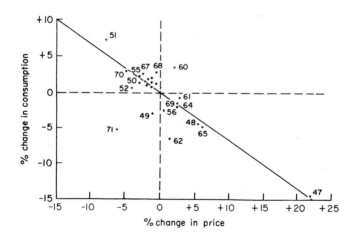

Fig. 27.3   Comparison of annual change in 'corrected' price and annual change in consumption by men, 1946-71.
Note: Each point on the graph represents one year. The line is the least squares regression line for annual consumption change on price change, excluding the years 1962 and 1971 (r = −0.91, P<0.001). The unlabelled points bunched in the upper left quadrant represent the years 1953, 1954, 1957, 1958, 1959, 1963, and 1966.

179

1967). The elasticity of the demand for a product is the per cent change in consumption that results from a one per cent change in price. A product has unit elasticity when a one per cent change in price causes a one per cent change in consumption. Products for which the elasticity exceeds one have 'elastic' demands. For such products a rise in price depresses sales so much that total expenditure on the product is less than it was at the lower price, while a drop in price increases total expenditure. On the other hand, products with an elasticity less than unity have 'inelastic' demands. For these products a rise in price reduces consumption proportionately less than the price increase so that total expenditure is increased. This is the case with cigarettes. The regression coefficients for consumption change on price change (−0.50 to −0.66, Table 27.2) are an index of elasticity. They indicate that for every one per cent rise in 'corrected' price, consumption fell by about 0.6 per cent. This analysis shows, therefore, that the demand for cigarettes is 'inelastic'. Economic studies have shown that food and necessities that have no adequate substitute tend to have 'inelastic' demands while luxuries and items that are easily substituted have 'elastic' demands (Dorfman, 1964). The low elasticity of the demand for cigarettes is a measure of dependence on them.

In their analysis of consumer behaviour in the United Kingdom between 1920 and 1938 the Department of Applied Economics at Cambridge (Stone, 1954) found the elasticity for tobacco products as a whole to be about −0.5. This finding of an 'inelastic' demand for cigarettes is in accordance with the present analysis. The slightly lower figure of the Cambridge study may be due to a number of facts. First, it refers to all tobacco products rather than to cigarettes alone. Secondly, their analysis was not confined to consumption by men. Also, compared with the post-war period, price fluctuations over the pre-war period were very small.

Other anti-smoking influences

It is just possible that the major change after 1949 of the intercept of the curve for consumption on 'corrected' price (Fig. 27.2) was an early influence of the evidence linking smoking with lung cancer. This is very tentative because the first solid report of the association with cancer was a year later, in 1950 (Doll and Hill, 1950).

The data of this study suggest that the two Royal College of Physicians' reports greatly depressed consumption. Both 1962 and 1971 produced marked atypical changes in slope between years in Figure 27.2. In 1962 the rise in 'corrected' price of 0.74 old pence per 20 cigarettes (Table 27.1) would, according to the regression coefficient of 32.23 (Table 27.2), be expected to have reduced consumption by 28.29 (38.23 × 0.74) to 3,982 per head per year instead of the actual figure of 3,750 for that year. The excess drop in consumption (equivalent to what would be expected to result from a 'corrected' price rise of 6.07 old pence for 20 cigarettes) is almost certainly attributable to the Royal College of Physicians' report. In the same way the 1971 report was associated with an excess drop over expected change in consumption equivalent to a 'corrected' price rise of 8.63 old pence per 20 cigarettes. Furthermore, contrary to what is usually said, the figures suggest that the change in intercept associated with the 1962 report was preserved until 1967 (Fig. 27.2), indicating more than a transient effect. It remains to be seen whether the effect of the 1971 report is more or less durable. As is the case with price increases, it is not possible to say from the present data whether the effect has been to make established smokers reduce or stop smoking or to lower recruitment to smoking.

There is no evidence from these data that the ban on cigarette advertising on television in August 1965 had any effect whatsoever. It could be, however, that there was an effect but that it was masked by the vigorous intensification of coupon promotion and other schemes with which manufacturers countered this move by the government.

Implications for smoking control

The first essential in the planning of any programme is to settle on the objectives. It is suggested here that to seek the eventual elimination of all forms of smoking is too extreme. Rather than anti-smoking the aim should be towards achieving acceptably safe controlled smoking. This would still require the virtual exclusion of cigarette smoking. Most smokers are simply unable to smoke cigarettes in a controlled non-dependent manner. There are two reasons for this. First, the rapid absorption through the lungs of nicotine from inhaled cigarette smoke mimics the effect of a series of small intravenous injections. Secondly, the ease of smoking cigarettes in many situations allows a frequency of use that almost invites dependence. These dangers are minimised in the case of pipe or large cigar smoking, provided the smoke is alkaline so as to allow slower absorption of nicotine through the buccal and nasal mucosa in a manner that is less likely to produce dependence.

Current interest in the development of a safe cigarette is to some extent misguided. To be completely safe, cigarette smoke would have to be not only carcinogen-free but free of nicotine and carbon monoxide as well. A nicotine-free cigarette would be unacceptable to most smokers, and carbon monoxide absorption can be reduced only by not inhaling. Cigarettes with a low tar content are no doubt safer but the position with low nicotine cigarettes is questionable. It is possible that they may even be more dangerous for established smokers who will tend to puff at them harder and more frequently to obtain their usual dose of nicotine.

The goal of acceptably safe controlled smoking would therefore require the virtual elimination of cigarette smoking in favour of pipes and cigars above a certain weight and at a price that would place them in the class of small luxuries. This could be achieved by selectively applying the price disincentive to cigarettes while adopting a more lenient approach to pipe and large cigar smoking. By leaving pipes and cigars as available substitutes the chances of troublesome cigarette black-marketeering would be reduced.

A feasible programme would be to increase tobacco tax selectively so as to raise the 'basic' price of cigarettes by about ten per cent a year. At this rate it would take 12 years for the cost of 20 cigarettes to reach £1. This rate of increase might need to be accelerated if the gearing to inflation or disposable income became substantially altered. This is not as harsh as it appears. There are certainly precedents for price rises of this order. In terms of proportion of disposable income, people in 1948 were paying for 20 standard plain cigarettes the 1971 equivalent of 13s. 7d. (68p) as opposed to what people in 1971 were actually paying, namely 6s. 2d. (31p). With regular price increases of this order it is likely that the elasticity of the demand for cigarettes would gradually climb above unity as cigarettes assumed the characteristics of luxury products. At this stage further price rises would become even more potent depressors of consumption. During such a programme the revenue obtained from tobacco tax would increase despite the drop in consumption, at least for as long as the elasticity of the demand for cigarettes remained below one.

With selective taxation along the lines suggested coupled to health education and other measures geared more towards achieving acceptably safe, controlled, non-dependent, non-inhaled puffing of alkaline smoke from pipes or large cigars, it is likely that dangerous cigarette smoking could be virtually eliminated within a decade.

28 Absorption by non-smokers of carbon monoxide from room air polluted by tobacco smoke*

M. A. H. RUSSELL, P. V. COLE and E. BROWN

Summary

Twenty subjects spent a mean of 78 minutes seated in an unventilated smoke-filled room of approximately $43m^3$ (15 × 12 × 8 ft). The smoke was produced by burning or smoking 80 cigarettes and two cigars. The average ambient carbon monoxide (CO) concentration was 38 ppm. Blood samples taken before and after the exposure showed an increase in carboxyhaemoglobin (COHb) in all subjects without exception (P < .001). The COHb of the 12 non-smokers increased from a mean of 1.6 to 2.6 per cent (P < .001), while the six cigarette smokers, all inhalers, besides having significantly higher initial levels (P < .001) also showed a greater increase from a mean of 5.9 to 9.6 per cent (P < .001). The two cigar smokers, one an inhaler and the other a non-inhaler, showed respective COHb changes similar to the cigarette smokers and non-smokers. The mean increase of one per cent COHb among the non-smokers was similar to the mean increase for the smokers of 0.7 per cent for each cigarette smoked, suggesting that the amount of CO which the non-smokers absorbed by passive smoking was about the same as would be expected if they had actively smoked and inhaled one cigarette.

Introduction

The level of venous blood carboxyhaemoglobin (COHb) in humans depends mainly on the rate of endogenous carbon monoxide (CO) production, the concentration of exogenous CO in the inspired air and alveolar ventilation (Coburn et al., 1965). Tobacco smoke contains as much as five per cent CO and smoking increases blood COHb (Lawther and Commins, 1970; US Department of Health, Education and Welfare, 1972). Attention has recently been directed at the possibility that tobacco smoke may also be a source of

---

* First published in *Lancet,* Vol. 1, 1973, pp. 576–9.

CO contamination for non-smokers in the vicinity of smokers especially if the exposure is prolonged and occurs in poorly ventilated confined places (Srch, 1967; Harke, 1970; Godber, 1971). Persistently raised COHb levels may be hazardous to health (US Department of Health, Education and Welfare, 1972; Astrup, 1972). We have attempted to assess how much non-smokers are put at risk by unavoidable 'passive smoking' of air which has been polluted, not by themselves, but by smokers.

Material and methods

Twenty-one research and clerical colleagues volunteered to provide blood specimens before and after spending at least one hour in a smoke-filled room. The conditions were deliberately made worse than would be likely to be encountered in natural social situations. The experimental room was approximately 43 m^3 (15 × 12 × 8 ft). Ventilators were switched off and all windows closed. Before subjects entered the room it was 'smoked up' by leaving 30 cigarettes (Piccadilly tipped) to burn in ashtrays. During the experiment the smokers smoked 32 cigarettes and two cigars; a further 18 cigarettes were left to burn in ashtrays. During the average time of 78 minutes spent in the experimental room subjects remained seated in the same place. The exposure was extremely unpleasant causing eyes to burn and water. For most subjects it was worse than they could recall having tolerated on normal social occasions.

At 18 minutes and 53 minutes after the subjects had entered the room (mean entry for all subjects), samples of room air were collected at heights of two and five feet above floor level. Air samples were collected into special gas-sampling bags (Hawkins, 1967) and analysed for CO with a Hartmann and Braun infra-red analyser (URAS 2). The zero point of the instrument was set with 0^2–free nitrogen and the span with 200 ppm CO in air (Rank Precision Industries). All samples were dried with magnesium perchlorate. The CO concentration of the first two samples was 37.0 ppm (2 ft) and 32.5 ppm (5 ft). For the second two samples, it was 41.8 (2 ft) and 41.3 (5 ft) giving an approximate average for the experiment of 38.2 ppm.

Venous blood samples were collected into heparinised syringes at an average of ten minutes before entry and 12 minutes after leaving the experimental room. The syringes were capped and stored in ice. The analysis for COHb was done on the same day using an IL 182 CO-Oximeter. Accuracy of this method was checked by comparison with the spectrophotometric method of Commins and Lawther (Commins and Lawther 1965; Lily et al., 1972). The correlation between the two methods were .99 for 33 specimens over the range of 0–11.7 per cent COHb. The

184

reproductibility was checked by taking four measurements of each of four specimens which gave the following means ± SE; 0.92% ± .03, 3.58% ± .03, 5.6% ± 0, 8.88% ± .05. Thus over the range employed the 95 per cent confidence limits of the reproductibility of the CO-Oximeter lie within 0.1 per cent COHb.

Results

The initial COHb levels (see Table 28.1 and Figure 28.1) were much higher in the smokers (mean 5.9 per cent) than in the non-smokers (mean 1.6 per cent) and the difference is statistically significant (t = 5.8, df = 17, P < .001). The initial COHb level of individual smokers was related to their usual cigarette consumption (r = .80, P < .05) and to the number of cigarettes smoked on the morning before the experiment (r = .79, P < .05).

After the experimental exposure, COHb was increased in all subjects without exception (t = 5.01, df = 17, P < .001). The COHb of non-smokers increased from the mean of 1.6 to 2.6 per cent (t = 5.9, df = 11, P < .001), while the smokers showed a substantially larger increase from a mean of 5.9 to 9.6 per cent. The greater mean increase of the smokers compared with the non-smokers (3.6 vs. 1.03 per cent) is statistically significant (t = 5.1, df = 16, P < .001). Among the smokers the rise in COHb was only modestly, but not significantly, related to the number of cigarettes smoked during the experiment (r = .55, P > .1) but there was a stronger relation to the length of time spent in the experimental room (r = .85, P < .05). Surprisingly the duration of exposure in the experimental room did not emerge as a significant factor determining the variation in COHb rise in the case of the non-smokers (r = −.38, n.s.).

The average rise in COHb for each smoker per cigarette smoked during the experiment was 0.7 per cent COHb (range 0.31–0.97, SD.24; see Figure 28.2). This is about the same as the mean increase of 1.03 per cent COHb for the non-smokers and suggests that the amount of CO that the non-smokers absorbed by passive smoking was roughly equivalent to the amount taken in by the smokers from one cigarette.

Discussion

The results indicate unequivocally that in circumstances of poor ventilation non-smokers do absorb CO from tobacco smoke produced when other people smoke. The rise in blood COHb levels of these 12 non-smokers from a mean of 1.6 to 2.6 per cent after an average of 79 minutes exposure to smoke-filled room-air containing about 38 ppm of CO accords well with two similar studies that are to be found in the German literature. In one (Srch, 1967), the smoking of ten cigarettes over a period of 62 minutes in an enclosed car produced a CO level of 90 ppm and caused the COHb of two non-smokers to increase from two to five per cent, while in the other (Harke, 1970) the levels of seven non-smokers increased from a mean of 0.9 to 2.1 per cent after they had spent about 90 minutes in a smoke-filled room containing 30 ppm of CO.

We have shown that the average COHb rise in smokers attributable to each cigarette smoked is about 0.7 per cent, which suggests that, in these admittedly extreme experimental circumstances, the amount of CO that the non-smokers absorbed by passive smoking was about the same as would be expected if they had actively smoked and inhaled one cigarette. It was also of the same order as a London taxi driver takes in from traffic pollution during a whole day of driving (mean COHb levels for non-smoking day drivers versus night drivers: 2.31 versus 1.04 per cent) (Jones et al., 1972) and similar to that absorbed by London policemen after three hours of point duty (Lawther and Commins, 1970).

A puzzling result was the absence among the non-smokers of a significant relation between the amount of CO absorbed and the duration of exposure. This is unlikely to have been due to a plateau effect as even by the end of the experiment their COHb levels were still well below the saturation level (approximately 5.5 per cent for the 38 ppm of CO in the room; US National Air Pollution Control Administration, 1970). Apart from the individual factors such as differences in pulmonary ventilation, part of the explanation may be accounted for by local variations in CO concentration in different parts of the room. It has been shown that the air in the vicinity of a smoker can show transient peaks exceeding 90 ppm (Lawther and Commins, 1970). The exceptionally large increase in COHb in one non-smoker (subject 18) could possibly be accounted for by the fact that he was sitting in the most smoky part of the room, between the two cigar smokers.

In the case of the smokers it is difficult to explain why the length of time spent in the experimental room had a stronger relation to the rise in COHb level than did the number of cigarettes smoked during the experiment. The COHb level of all the smokers ended up well above the 5.5 per cent equilibrium saturation level for the CO in the room. Above this level the rise in COHb could only have been mediated by smoking; indeed, without smoking it would gradually fall. Part of the explanation may lie in variation in the degree of inhalation. They were reluctant to smoke as much as they did and did so only because they had been so instructed. The smokers who followed the instructions conscientiously and smoked more may have consequently inhaled less, while those who disregarded the instructions may have smoked less but continued to inhale as usual.

186

Because there were only two, the cigar smokers were not used for the analysis. However, they do demonstrate that as far as CO is concerned a cigar smoker who inhales differs little from cigarette smokers, while the non-inhaler had COHb levels identical with the non-smokers, confirming the fact that little absorption of CO takes place through the buccal mucosa (US Dept. of Health, Education and Welfare, 1972).

The experimental conditions were somewhat extreme. This degree of tobacco smoke pollution is unlikely to be encountered with any frequency in 'natural' social situations. However, the exposure time was short compared with some social situations. Even with slightly better ventilation three or four hours in a smoky car or pub would almost certainly involve a non-smoker in significant passive smoking. Further work is indicated in more natural settings. Though the amounts of CO absorbed by passive smoking are very small compared with active smoking, there may well be appreciable long-term negative health consequences (US Dept. of Health, Education and Welfare, 1972; Astrup, 1972). Evidence is also beginning to accrue that subtle perceptual abilities such as visual acuity, brightness threshold, and time interval discrimination may be temporarily impaired by absorption of small amounts of CO at blood COHb levels as low as three per cent (Beard and Grandstaff, 1970), and three of the non-smokers in the present experiment reached this level. Finally there is suggestive evidence that passive smoking may result in absorption of other potentially hazardous components of tobacco smoke, for example, tar, nicotine, 3.4-benzpyrene and oxides of nitrogen (NO, NO_2), (US National Air Pollution Control Administration, 1970). It seems, therefore, that in addition to discomfort, occasional allergic reactions, nasal and conjunctival irritation, a small but real health risk is another potential consequence of passive smoking. This is an order of risk that smokers are prepared to take many times a day, but insignificant though it may be compared with active smoking, it is a risk that many non-smokers may wish to avoid. They should at least have a choice.

Table 28·1

Changes in COHb levels after an average of 78 minutes in a smoky room containing about 38 ppm CO

Smoking status	Subject	Sex	Age	Usual tobacco consumption (cigarettes per day)	Amount smoked in morning before experiment (no. of cigarettes)	Amount smoked during experiment (no. of cigarettes)	Time spent in experimental room (minutes)	Blood COHb Levels		
								Before %	After %	Difference %
	1	F	22	25	8	6	86	7.2	12.2	+5.0
	2	F	28	40	12	7	76	6.8	9.0	+2.2
Cigarette	3	F	41	40	10	3	55	10.3	11.9	+1.6
smokers	4	F	27	25	5	7	81	4.1	9.0	+4.9
n=7	5	M	27	15	3	6	100	2.6	7.7	+5.1
	6	M	22	15	6	3	65	4.7	7.6	+2.9
	7 a	F	25	25	5	–	–	5.8	–	–
				Mean 26 SD 10.3	Mean 7 SD 3 2	Mean 5.3 SD 1.9	Mean 77 SD 16.2	Mean 5.9 SD 2.6	Mean 9.6 SD 1.8	Mean 3.6 SD 1.5

	Subject	Sex	Age	3 cigars Occasional cigar	1 cigar None	1 cigar 1 cigar				
Cigar smokers n=2	8	M	44				79	6.5	8.4	+1.9
	9b	M	29				60	1.4	2.3	+0.9
	10	F	34				72	1.0	2.7	+1.7
	11	F	35				72	0.9	1.7	+0.8
	12	F	24				102	1.7	2.6	+0.9
	13	M	30				75	2.1	3.2	+1.1
	14	M	36	N	N	N	101	1.9	2.2	+0.3
	15	M	40	O	O	O	52	0.7	1.8	+1.1
	16	M	29	N	N	N	63	2.2	3.3	+1.1
Non smokers n=12	17	M	26	E	E	E	99	0.9	2.4	+1.5
	18	M	22				77	1.8	4.2	+2.4
	19	M	24				63	2.2	2.6	+0.4
	20	M	34				68	1.8	2.6	+0.8
	21	M	29				104	2.1	2.4	+0.3
							Mean 79	Mean 1.6	Mean 2.6	Mean 1.03
							SD 17.9	SD 0.6	SD 0.7	SD 0.6

a This subject dropped out due to faintness after the initial blood specimen was taken.
b All the smokers were habitual inhalers with the exception of subject 9.

189

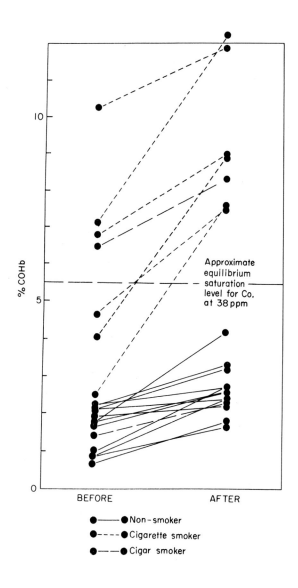

Fig. 28.1   Changes in blood COHb after spending a mean of 78 minutes in a smoke-filled room containing a mean of 38 ppm CO.

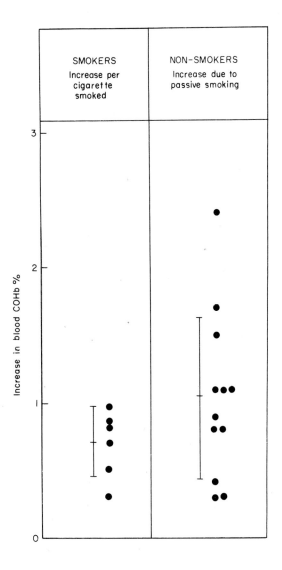

Fig. 28.2 Increase in COHb levels of non-smokers due to 'passive smoking' compared with increase in smokers per cigarette smoked. Both smokers and non-smokers spent an average of 78 minutes in the same smoky room containing a mean of 38 ppm CO. Lines indicate the means ± 1 SD. The difference between the means is not significant.

29 Comparison of effect on tobacco consumption and carbon monoxide absorption of changing to high and low nicotine cigarettes*

M. A. H. RUSSELL, C. WILSON, U. A. PATEL, P. V. COLE, C. FEYERABEND

Summary

In ten sedentary workers, smoking as they felt inclined over a five-hour period in the middle of a typical working day, changing to low nicotine cigarettes (< 0.3 mg) caused an increase in the number and weight of cigarettes smoked, while changing to high nicotine cigarettes (3.2 mg) caused a decrease (P < 0.01). When smoking the usual brand the average blood carboxyhaemoglobin (COHb) increased 1.78 per cent (from 6.38 per cent to 8.16 per cent). But on changing to either high or low nicotine cigarettes the COHb levels instead of increasing, tended to fall (P < 0.01). The average fall of 0.34 per cent while smoking low nicotine cigarettes was due to the low carbon monoxide (CO) yield of these cigarettes, while the fall of 1.04 per cent when smoking high nicotine cigarettes was atributable to reduced consumption. The findings support the view that smoking behaviour is modified to regulate nicotine intake. Besides having low tar and CO yields, the least harmful cigarettes for heavy smokers may be those with a high, rather than low, nicotine yield.

Introduction

On 11 April 1973 the Government published for the first time the tar and nicotine yields of 101 brands of cigarette sold in the United Kingdom (DHSS 1973; *Lancet* 1973). Behind the publication of this 'league table' lies the assumption that it is less hazardous to smoke cigarettes with a low yield of tar and nicotine (Royal College of Physicians, 1971; Wynder, 1972). Recently we have shown that cigarettes also vary in their carbon monoxide (CO) yield (Russell et al., 1973a). This suggests that any consideration of a cigarette's degree of hazard is incomplete without information about its CO yield, and

---

* First published in the *British Medical Journal*, Vol. 4, 1973, pp. 512–6.

that CO yield should be added to official publications of tar and nicotine yield.

Safer though it may be to take in less nicotine, tar, and CO, to what extent is this achieved by changing to a low nicotine cigarette? The information available is scanty and conflicting. It has, for instance, been clearly shown in two independent studies (Ashton et al., 1970; Frith, 1971) that smokers unconsciously modified their puff rate to regulate their nicotine intake. When smoking a high nicotine cigarette they puffed less often and when smoking a low nicotine cigarette they increased their puff rate and thus compensated for the low nicotine yield. A change to cigarettes of lower nicotine yield, however, does not seem to lead to increased consumption in terms of the number smoked per day (Waingrow and Horn, 1968), nor does reducing the nicotine yield by cutting cigarettes to half length cause a compensatory increase in the number smoked (Goldfarb and Jarvik, 1972). There is, however, some evidence that as the nicotine content of the cigarette is increased the number smoked declines (Goldfarb et al., 1970).

The main aim of this study was to attempt to resolve the question of the role of nicotine yield as a determinant of the amount of cigarettes smoked. If lowering the nicotine yield does indeed give rise to a compensatory increase in inhalation with consequent increased absorption of tar and CO, or if raising the nicotine yield lowers the amount smoked, the assumption that low nicotine cigarettes are less hazardous would need to be re-examined (Russell, 1972). It would then become necessary to focus on the ratio of the nicotine yield to the tar and CO yield and to consider the possibility that the safer cigarette might be the one with a high nicotine yield but low tar and CO yield.

We have also attempted to verify predictions arising out of the findings of previous work (Russell et al., 1973a) which indicated that the smoking frequency would have to be extremely high for the COHb level to increase appreciably when smoking cigarettes with a low CO yield. For example, smokers with blood COHb levels in the region of 6–7 per cent would have to smoke at least one of these cigarettes every 20 minutes just to maintain the same level.

Methods

Ten clerical and social workers volunteered to take part in the experiment. All were regular cigarette smokers who said that they inhaled deeply. Cigarette consumption was studied over four five-hour periods, from mid-morning to mid-afternoon, on four separate working days; two consecutive days of one week and the same two days of the following week. On the first day of each week's dyad the subjects smoked their usual brand of cigarette and on the

Table 29.1

Changes in cigarette consumption of sedentary workers over five-hour period of smoking usual, low nicotine, and high nicotine cigarettes

Subjects			Usual Cigarettes Smoked			Cigarette Consumption over Five-hour Period							
						First Week				Second Week			
						Usual Brand (Day 1)		Experimental Brand (Day 2)		Usual Brand (Day 1)		Experimental Brand (Day 2)	
No.	Sex	Age	Brand	Nicotine Yield (mg)	No./day	No.	Weight (gg)	No.	Weight (gg)	No.	Weight (gg)	No.	Weight (gg)
1	M	25	Player's No. 6 Filter	1.2	25	9	3.97	9*	4.97	13	5.55	8†	5.73
2	M	19	Embassy Filter	1.3	30	9	6.28	15*	8.87	8	5.46	7†	6.07
3	F	20	Embassy Filter	1.3	17	6	3.60	8*	4.02	4	2.64	4†	2.35
4	F	23	Gitanes Caporal Filter	1.4	35	12	7.99	13*	6.50	16	9.84	9†	5.14
5	F	22	Embassy Filter	1.3	30	19	10.32	17*	8.18	16	8.35	5†	1.78
6	M	25	Rothman's King Size	1.4	35	12	9.14	6†	3.66	12	8.80	15*	8.22
7	M	63	Player's Weights Plain	1.6	18	10	5.31	7†	5.29	11	6.14	14*	7.18
8	F	26	Player's Gold Leaf	1.5	35	10	6.26	8†	4.59	7	3.74	15*	7.66
9	F	48	Player's No. 6 Filter	1.2	25	6	2.83	5†	3.02	9	3.96	10*	5.36
10	F	29	Player's No. 6 Filter	1.2	22	12	5.08	8†	4.22	12	4.78	9*	4.25
Mean±S.D.		30±14.2		1.34±0.13	27.2±6.86	10.5±3.7	6.08±2.44			10.8±3.9	5.93±2.37		

* Low nicotine cigarette.
† High nicotine cigarette.

194

Table 29.2
Changes in COHb levels in sedentary workers before and after five-hour period of smoking usual, low nicotine, and high nicotine cigarettes

Blood Carboxyhaemoglobin Levels (%)

Subjects			First Week						Second Week					
			Usual Brand (Day 1)			Experimental Brand (Day 2)			Usual Brand (Day 1)			Experimental Brand (Day 2)		
No.	Sex	Age	Before	After	Difference	Before	After	Difference	Before	After	Difference	Before	After	Difference
1	M	25	6.2	9.0	+2.8	7.0	7.3*	+0.3	8.2	10·8	+2.6	8.0	‡ †	
2	M	19	6.1	8.7	+2.6	7.4	7.3*	−0.1	8.0	9.7	+1.7	8.3	6.9†	−1.4
3	F	20	3.7	4.3	+0.6	4.0	3.9*	−0.1	5.6	4.9	−0.7	4.8	3.7†	−1.1
4	F	23	5.0	9.5	+4.5	7.8	6.5*	−1.3	6.9	13·0	+6.1	6.7	7.2†	+0.5
5	F	22	5.2	9.1	+3.9	6.3	8.0*	+1.7	3.9	8.8	+4.9	4.3	2.8†	−1.5
6	M	25	5.5	7.9	+2.4	4.7	3.9†	−0.8	6.4	8.4	+2.0	6.2	7.4*	+1.2
7	M	63	7.3	9.2	+1.9	7.1	6.5†	−0.6	7.6	9.1	+1.5	7.7	7.6*	−0.1
8	F	26	4.6	6.3	+1.7	3.4	4.0†	+0.6	5.1	5.0	−0.1	4.8	5.1*	+0.3
9	F	48	10.2	9.3	−0.9	10.3	6.7†	−3.6	11.4	8.6	−2.8	11.2	6.2*	−5.0
10	F	29	5.0	6.6	+1.6	5.6	4.1†	−1.5	5.6	5.0	−0.6	2.6	‡ *	
Mean ± S.D.		30 ± 14.2	5.88±1.81	7.99±1.72	2.11±1.55				6.87±2.09	8.33±2.68	1.46±2.67			

*Low nicotine cigarette.
†High nicotine cigarette.
‡Blood specimen clotted.

second day they smoked either a high or a low nicotine cigarette. Half the subjects were randomly assigned to smoke the low nicotine cigarette on the first week and the high nicotine cigarette on the second week; with the other half this order was reversed (see Tables 29.1 and 29.2). The high nicotine cigarette used was Capstan Full Strength (tar 38 mg, nicotine 3.2 mg), and the low nicotine cigarette was Silk Cut Extra Mild (tar 4 mg, nicotine < 0.3 mg). These two cigarettes occupy the top and bottom positions of the current tar and nicotine 'league table' (DHSS, 1973; *Lancet, 1973*). The low nicotine cigarette was filter tipped but the high nicotine one was plain.

For each of the five-hour periods studied subjects were given an adequate supply of the appropriate brand of cigarette with instructions not to offer them to others and to smoke as much or as little as they felt inclined, but only from the cigarettes supplied. We estimated the number of cigarettes smoked by subtracting the remaining cigarettes from the number in the full packets which were supplied. Subjects also stored their cigarette ends and this provided an additional check on the number smoked and enabled consumption to be calculated in terms of the weight of cigarettes burned up in the five-hour study period.

Venous blood was taken before and after each five-hour period. No restrictions were placed on smoking on the morning before the experiment, but to avoid error due to variation in time-span between the last cigarette and collection of the blood sample subjects were required to smoke a cigarette immediately before each blood sample, which was then taken about three minutes after completion of that cigarette. The blood samples were collected in heparinised syringes which were capped and stored in a refrigerator. The analysis for COHb was done on the same day with an IL 182 CO-Oximeter. This is an accurate method with reproducibility having 95 per cent confidence limits within 0.1 per cent COHb (Russell et al., 1973b).

Visual analogue scales (Aitken, 1969) were used for comparing the different brands of cigarette on subjective ratings of 'satisfaction,' 'strength,' and 'taste evaluation'. Subjects indicated their ratings by making a mark at the appropriate point on a series of 100-mm horizontal lines between two extremes. Average test-retest reliability for all scales between morning and afternoon ratings of the usual brand of cigarette was satisfactory (r = 0.91). Statistical analysis was by Student's *t* test.

Results

Changes in number of cigarettes smoked

When subjects were smoking their usual brand of cigarette the number

196

smoked over the five-hour experimental period was fairly consistent from one week to the next (r = 0.75; P < 0.02), the means for the first and second week being 10.5 and 10.8 respectively (Table 29.1). On changing to low nicotine cigarettes the numbers smoked increased from a mean of 10.6 (for the usual brand) to 12.5 (Table 29.3) but this increase is not statistically significant (t = 1.8; D.F. = 9). On changing to high nicotine cigarettes, however, there was a 38 per cent decrease from a mean of 10.7 to 6.7 (t = 3.8; D.F. = 9; P <0.01). The difference is even more striking when the average number smoked of the low and high nicotine cigarettes is compared (12.5 v. 6.7; t = 5.3; D.F. = 9; P < 0.001).

Changes in weight of cigarettes smoked

The differences between brands in the weight of cigarettes smoked in the five-hour period are of a similar pattern to the differences in numbers smoked (Tables 29.1 and 29.3). There was great consistency between the first and second weeks in the weight smoked of the usual brand, the respective means being 6.08 g and 5.93 g (r = 0.81; P < 0.01). The tendency to smoke slightly more of the low nicotine cigarettes was not statistically significant, but the tendency to smoke less of the high nicotine cigarettes compared with the usual brand was significant (4.19 g v. 6.04 g; t = 2.2; D.F. = 9; P < 0.05). The difference in the weight smoked of low and high nicotine cigarettes was also significant (6.52 g; v. 4.19 g; t = 3.6; D.F. = 9; P < 0.01).

COHb changes

The average initial COHb level over all four days was 6.48 per cent ($\pm$ 2.05 S.D.). It was fairly consistent between the four days (see Tables 29.2 and 29.3: r = 0.78 to 0.93; P < 0.01). When the subjects were smoking their usual cigarettes the percentage of COHb showed a mean increase of 1.78, from 6.38 per cent to 8.16 per cent, over the five-hour smoking period. This increase is statistically significant (t = 3.7; D.F. = 19; P < 0.005; first and second week combined). The COHb increase was also fairly consistent from the first to the second week (mean 2.11 per cent v. 1.46 per cent; r = 0.97; P < 0.001). In contrast to the usual brand, when smoking either high or low nicotine cigarettes the COHb levels decreased rather than increased over the five-hour smoking period (Table 29.3). On the low nicotine cigarette there was a fall of 0.34 per cent, which differed significantly from the increase on the usual brand (t = 3.5; D.F. = 8; P < 0.01), while on the high nicotine cigarette the fall of 1.04 per cent also differed significantly from the increase on the usual brand (t = 4.9; D.F. = 8; P < 0.01). The difference in the COHb decreases on the high and low nicotine cigarettes is not statistically significant.

Table 29.3
Average consumption and COHb changes over five-hour period of smoking usual, low nicotine, and high nicotine cigarettes

Brand of Cigarette	Amount Smoked in Five Hours (Mean ± S.D.)		Blood Carboxyhaemoglobin Levels (%) (Mean ± S.D.)		
	No. of Cigarettes	Weight (g)	Before	After	Difference
Usual	10.6 ± 3.6	5.96 ± 2.38	6.23 ± 2.09	7.67 ± 2.04	+1.44 ± 2.21
Silk Cut Extra Mild (nicotine < 0.3 mg)	12.5 ± 3.2	6.52 ± 1.76	6.93* ± 2.06	6.59* ± 1.34	−0.34* ± 1.94
Usual	10.7 ± 3.9	6.04 ± 2.44	6.52 ± 1.95	8.65 ± 2.35	+2.13 ± 2.15
Capstan Full Strength (nicotine 3.2 mg)	6.7 ± 1.6	4.19 ± 1.45	6.13* ± 2.19	5.09* ± 1.70	−1.04* ± 1.25

* Mean of nine subjects. Other means ± 1 S.D. are derived from 10 subjects.

Mean values for usual brand of cigarette differ slightly from those in Tables 29.1 and 29.2. Values shown here are split across first and second weeks to make a more valid comparison with cross-over 'experimental' cigarettes. Thus 'experimental' cigarettes are compared with 'usual' cigarette values of preceding day.

In the case of the usual brand of cigarette there was a positive relation between COHb increase over five-hours and the amount smoked during this period both in terms of the number of cigarettes smoked (r = 0.71; P < 0.01) and the weight of cigarettes smoked (r = 0.78; P < 0.01). However, there was no such association when smoking either the high or the low nicotine cigarettes.

Subjective ratings of cigarette brands

The usual brand of cigarette was rated before and after the five-hour smoking period on the first day, and after the smoking period on each of the subsequent days (Fig. 29.1) The values shown are therefore the means of five ratings. The high and low nicotine cigarettes were rated only once, immediately after the five-hour period in which they were smoked. On average the usual cigarettes tasted 'very good,' were 'very satisfying,' and were neither 'too strong' nor 'too weak'. When compared with the usual brand the low nicotine cigarette was much 'too weak' (P < 0.001) and not at all 'satisfying' (P < 0.001) or 'good tasting' (P < 0.001); the high nicotine cigarette, on the other hand, was moderately 'satisfying' (P < 0.02) and 'good tasting' (not significant) despite being far 'too strong' (P < 0.01).

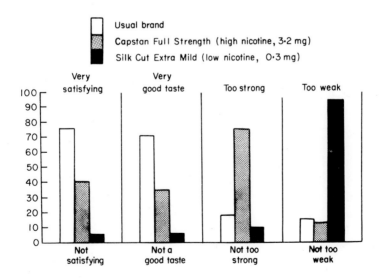

Fig. 29.1 Average subjective ratings of different cigarette brands. See text for significance of differences.

199

Prediction of COHb changes with periodic smoking

Data from a previous study (Russell et al., 1973a) were subjected to further analysis to predict and explain the COHb changes of the present study. The regression of COHb level on COHb fall in 20 minutes provides estimates of the expected COHb fall over 20 minutes at rest for the range of COHb levels often found in smokers (see Table 29.4). The estimated half life for COHb based on the regression equation is two to two and a half hours. The average initial COHb level for all subjects on all four days of the present study was 6.48 per cent (see above). The estimated decline over 20 minutes for this initial level is 0.61 per cent. Since the smoking of a single Silk Cut Extra Mild cigarette produces an average COHb increase of only 0.64 per cent (Russell et al., 1973b), it follows that on average the subjects would have to smoke about one such cigarette every 20 minutes – that is, 15 cigarettes in the five-hour smoking period – to maintain the same COHb level (see Fig. 29.2). In those smoking more than 15 an increase would be expected, while in those smoking fewer than 15 there should be a decrease. This is more or less what happened (see Tables 29.1 and 29.2). Those subjects (Nos. 2, 5, 6, and 8) who smoked 15 or more of the low nicotine cigarettes (Silk Cut Extra Mild) in five hours tended to maintain or increase their COHb while the only substantial falls occurred in those who smoked fewer cigarettes.

Table 29.4
Pattern of decline in blood COHb level while sitting and not smoking for 20 minutes

Blood COHb level (%)	3	4	5	6	7	8	9	10	11
Expected fall in 20 min (%)		0.31	0.40	0.48	0.57	0.66	0.75	0.83	0.92	1.00

Based on data from 22 subjects of a previous study (Russell et al., 1973b). Regression equation for COHb level on fall in 20 min: $Y^1 = 0.09 \ X + 0.05$; $r = 0.65$; $P < 0.01$. Estimated half life for COHb based on this equation is two to two and a half hours.

There was even more concordance between the predictions and findings in the case of 'non-mild' cigarettes – that is, usual and high nicotine taken together. Average COHb increase after smoking a single non-mild cigarette was 1.27 per cent (mean of Embassy Filter = 1.45, and Player's No. 6 Filter = 1.09) (Russell et al., 1973b). Thus, very approximately it would need a smoking rate of about one cigarette every 40 minutes – seven to eight cigarettes in the five-hour smoking period — to offset the expected mean rate of COHb decrease for these subjects (1.17 per cent in 40 minutes; see Fig. 29.2). The findings (Tables 29.1 and 29.2) show this prediction to be well substantiated. Taking the values for both days on usual cigarettes together with the values for the high nicotine cigarette, of the 19 five-hour periods when eight or more cigarettes were smoked 16 were associated with an increase in COHb whereas there was a fall in COHb in nine out of 10 five-hour periods when less than eight cigarettes were smoked (P < 0.005, Fisher's exact test).

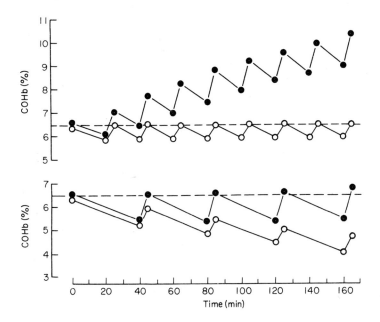

Fig. 29.2   Predicted pattern of COHb changes on smoking extra-mild (0–0) and non-mild (●—●) cigarettes at 20 min and 40 min intervals in subjects with a mean initial COHb level of 6.5 per cent (broken rule). Based on data from 22 subjects of a previous study (Russell et al., 1973b). Regression equation for COHb level on fall in 20 min: $Y^1 = 0.09 X + 0.05$; $r = 0.65$; $P < 0.01$. See text for mean increases in COHb per cigarette.

Discussion

The number of cigarettes smoked by this sample of sedentary workers smoking their usual brand of cigarettes during a five-hour period in the middle of a typical working day averaged 10.6 cigarettes of which 6.00 g was actually burned. The quantity smoked was fairly consistent between a given day of one week and the same day of the next week. When the subjects changed to smoking a low nicotine brand (Silk Cut Extra Mild) the amount smoked increased to a mean of 12.5 cigarettes (6.52 g burned) and when they changed to a high nicotine brand (Capstan Full Strength) the amount smoked decreased to a mean of 6.7 cigarettes (4.19 g burned). The tendency to increase consumption on changing to low nicotine cigarettes did not reach statistical significance but the tendency to reduce consumption of high nicotine cigarettes was statistically significant ($P < 0.01$). It is just possible that some of the difference in the number of cigarettes smoked between the usual and 'experimental' brands was due to the fact that they were smoked on different weekdays, but this would not have affected the highly significant difference ($P < 0.001$) in the amount smoked between the two 'experimental' brands (low nicotine and high nicotine) which were smoked on the same weekday.

The subjects were carefully instructed to smoke 'as they felt inclined'. The consistency from one week to the next when smoking the usual brand of cigarettes and the balanced cross-over design used for the smoking of the two 'experimental' brands make it extremely unlikely that the differences in the quantities smoked were due to anything other than differences in inclination to smoke different quantities of the different brands. Such differences in inclination could, however, have been due to differences in either palatability or nicotine yield. The fact that the subjects smoked more of the low nicotine cigarette which was rated very unfavourably and less of the high nicotine cigarette which was rated only moderately unfavourably suggests that the nicotine yield was the most important determinant of the changes in the quantity smoked. These findings therefore support those studies cited above (Ashton et al., 1970; Goldfarb et al., 1970; Frith, 1971) which indicate that regular smokers who inhale modify their smoking behaviour to regulate their nicotine intake.

Previous workers have always shown that the COHb level of smokers is at its lowest in the morning before smoking and that it tends to rise as subjects smoke throughout the day (Bowden and Woodhall, 1964; Goldsmith, 1970; US Dept. of Health, Education and Welfare, 1972). This pattern was repeated in the present study when subjects were smoking their usual brand of cigarettes. Over the five-hour period from mid-morning to mid-afternoon the average COHb percentage increased from 6.38 to 8.16 (Tables 29.2 and 29.3). But when the subjects changed to smoking either high nicotine or low nicotine cigarettes, instead of increasing, the COHb level tended to fall slightly. Compared with the average increase of 1.78 per cent when smoking

202

their usual cigarettes, there was an average decrease of 1.04 per cent when smoking high nicotine cigarettes (P < 0.01) and a decrease of 0.34 per cent when smoking the low nicotine cigarettes (P < 0.01). The fact that the COHb decreased on switching to high nicotine cigarettes can be accounted for by the reduction in the amount smoked. In the case of the low nicotine cigarettes, however, the decrease in COHb occurred despite an increase in the amount smoked and this is probably explained by the low CO yield of this brand of low nicotine cigarette (Russell et al., 1973a).

With knowledge gained from our previous study (Russell et al., 1973b) about the rate of decline of COHb in resting subjects and its dependence on the actual level of COHb, together with data on the very different increase in COHb produced by smoking 'non-mild' (Embassy Filter and Player's No. 6 Filter) as opposed to 'extra-mild' (Silk Cut Extra Mild) cigarettes, we were able to predict and explain the changes observed in the present study. Due to their low CO yield, the smoking of extra-mild cigarettes does not increase COHb appreciably even when smoked as heavily as one every 20 minutes – that is, about 50 a day (Fig. 29.2). On the other hand, with non-mild cigarettes this high smoking rate would produce a steady increase in COHb to the high levels (10–15 per cent) which occur in heavy smokers. It should be emphasised that these estimates, illustrating COHb fluctuations with smoking, apply only to subjects at rest. The overall tendency for COHb to rise with smoking would be very much less in more physically active subjects. The relation of COHb dynamics to exercise could partly account for the belief that the adverse effects on health of smoking and lack of exercise are synergistic or mutually enhancing. It also suggests that those who spend their evenings smoking heavily while slumped in an armchair for several hours before retiring are especially prone to prolonged exposure to raised COHb levels.

The COHb half life estimated from the regression equation in Table 29.4 was only two to two and a half hours. This is appreciably less than the generally accepted figure of three to four hours (US National Air Pollution Control Administration, 1970). This difference may be explained by the fact that previous determinations of COHb half life have been made after more prolonged exposures to inspired air CO. This allows more time for equilibration between COHb and extravascular sites such as myoglobin than is the case with the brief intermittent exposures to the far higher CO levels (two to five per cent) (Wynder and Hoffman, 1967) inhaled by tobacco smokers. Though each type of CO exposure may produce equivalent COHb levels, in the former case the COHb decline is due mainly to loss through the lungs while after the acute rise produced by a bout of smoking there may be an additional loss of CO from Hb to myoglobin.

It seems paradoxically to be the case that the two least hazardous cigarettes, at least in terms of CO exposure, are those at the top and bottom of the current tar and nicotine 'league table'. The low nicotine brand (Silk Cut Extra Mild) produces little rise in COHb levels because of its low CO yield, while the high nicotine yield of the other (Capstan Full Strength) so reduces consumption that again little rise in COHb is produced.

But what about overall safety? Apart from other factors such as the pH of the smoke, the sugar content, and method of curing the tobacco which are not the concern of this study, our findings suggest that for heavy smokers a cigarette would be less harmful if it combined the qualities of the low nicotine and the high nicotine brands by having a low tar and CO yield but a high, rather than low, nicotine yield.

The ideal of a cigarette with a low nicotine, low tar, and low CO yield is unfortunately not feasible for most smokers whose main reason for smoking is to obtain nicotine (Russell, 1971a). Besides the tendency for consumption to be increased, a low nicotine yield is unfortunately not feasible for most smokers. None of the 32 smokers in this study and our previous study (Russell et al., 1973b) was prepared to change permanently to the low nicotine brand (Silk Cut Extra Mild). On the other hand, a cigarette with a high nicotine yield would enable heavy smokers to curb their tobacco consumption, and harmfulness would be further reduced if, at the same time, the tar and CO yields were low.

At present a cigarette combining a high nicotine yield with a low tar and CO yield does not, so far as we know, exist. The correlation between the tar and nicotine yields of the cigarettes on the current 'league table' is high (0.96). To reduce tar yield without lowering the nicotine yield presents a challenge to cigarette technology but it is one which the skill and resources available are no doubt capable of meeting; especially if prompted by appropriate selective taxation.

30 Appraisal

One undoubted conclusion so far as the Unit itself is concerned must be that the smoking research group has during the relatively short space of its existence made it unthinkable that smoking research should not be represented within the Unit's spectrum of activities. The World Health Organisation with its emphasis on the 'combined approach' has done much to persuade researchers, clinicians and administrators of the many commonalities between drugs and alcohol, but nicotine is still not seen as one of the drugs that have to be combined into that approach – there is at every level a continued reluctance to admit smoking to full membership of the drug club. The experience of the Addiction Research Unit shows that some representation of research on smoking within a dependence research programme adds many awarenesses. Among the most fundamental contributions may be the different feeling tone which attaches to smoking as presenting a set of problems uncontaminated by our preconceptions relating to illegal drug use, or by the latent moral judgements which cluster around alcoholism. From the experimental point of view smoking may be an extremely convenient form of behaviour for setting up paradigms to study essential and general aspects of dependence.

An appraisal of these five papers on the smoking questions also points the reminder that any effective approach to a dependence problem must be at the individual as well as at the public health level, and both these complementary approaches must be underpinned by scientific knowledge which will come only from a range of disciplines as diverse as experimental psychology, economics, and biochemistry, to name but a few of the possible contributors.

The trial of aversion therapy, though preliminary and uncontrolled, indicates the manner in which a behavioural approach may be applied to smoking, and further controlled work along the same lines which is now awaiting publication has examined not only the practical value of such treatments but the theoretical implications for understanding of the learning processes which may be involved in such therapy. Work now in progress will examine parallel psychological treatments for alcoholism and smoking. The belief that investigation of therapies should by the same token be testing of theories as to the nature of dependence becomes more real. If dependence is a learning process it should be capable of dismantling by rational psychological treatments, and smoking may perhaps show the way.

The analysis of price relationships is in some ways parallel to the sustained concern in recent years of Toronto's Addiction Research Foundation with alcohol consumption and liquor price. The work of the group in Toronto is a prime example of social research having been addressed effectively and directly to issues of social policy. Any appraisal of this line of research must lead to the conclusion that there is work here for the professional economist to take further. And even the most guarded interpretation of this research would challenge the traditional notion of government that taxation is not a proper instrument of public health; men may perhaps be made healthy by taxation, even if not made moral by legislation. This research must also in the long term pose important questions for the planning of inter-disciplinary research. How is the economic expertise and the understanding of the subtleties of health data to be brought together? Perhaps indeed the reverential attitude to disciplinary co-operation deserves in this instance to be scrutinised rather critically – the economist, the designer of chemically safer cigarettes, the expert in dependence have the choice of being members of the same team, members of the same working party, or simply of reading each other's papers on the basis of catch-as-catch-can. Which is the preferred solution? Smoking research again forces the question.

The laboratory studies speak to a different range of complexities. That study of the role of nicotine in dependence must be crucial to understanding of cigarette smoking cannot now be doubted. Blood-nicotine assay has recently become feasible. But it is the balance between nicotine content, tar content and carbon monoxide yield which provides the interlocking puzzle for anyone who would hope to deal with health damage by making the cigarette less addictive and less damaging.

The conclusion of this appraisal might well be exactly that implied by the title of the first paper in this section: we come back to the notion that the effective contribution in such an area as dependence must very much imply the well devised research strategy rather than just one piece of research and then another, with disciplines striking only glancing blows.

206

THE RESEARCH POSITION

31   Introduction

The larger part of this book is devoted to presentation of the conventional end-product of research. The present section stands back and looks at what the business of research is actually about – the research position. The phrase hides, of course, a host of questions and only a few of them will be dealt with here.

The first two papers are short essays which focus on matters which concern the working life of any research unit. The business of research is the collection of facts and the honest and temperate extraction of the maximum of meaning from those facts, and here the statistician plays a vital role in the research group not only as technician but also as the friend and counsellor who is somewhat apart from the personalised involvements of other members of the group. Another matter bearing on the interpretation of the garnered facts is knowledge of what facts others have accumulated, and this implies an accurate and up-to-date acquaintance with the forever burgeoning literature. The essay by Peter Nicholls discusses the role of the statistician, and that by Maxine MacCafferty the role of the information scientist.

So much for an inward look at some important matters related to the functioning of a research unit. The research worker must also look outward, and in this regard he really faces in two general directions. On the one hand he must relate to the realities of the human problem down the road and be very careful not to set himself at too great and privileged distance from the human suffering and the sharply real social processes. In this regard Timothy Cook (as a social worker) and Alan Ogborne (a social scientist) have provided interesting complementary essays mutually sensitive to each other's positions.

And on the other hand, if the research worker does not have adequate communication with the decision makers and designers of government policy who are the potential consumers of the garnered facts, the research reports will have been written to no purpose and will do no more than gather dust on the library shelves. David Hawks therefore rounds off this section by a discussion of the relationship between social science and social policy.

32 Social research as a determinant of social policy*

DAVID HAWKS

Summary

An attempt is made to identify some of the constraints which limit the more effective meeting of social research and social policy. A system of public sponsorship for research which does not ensure its final application is an extravagance. The researcher's proclivity for independence, for academic freedom in the choice of his subject, his lack of public accountability, have served not only to ensure his immunity from interference, but have guaranteed his impotence. The policy maker contributes to the difficulty with expectations of science which may be unreal. A greater drawing together would be of benefit to everyone concerned.

Introduction

At conferences speakers tend either to enumerate the findings of research they have undertaken or else invoke the need for further research in areas of interest to them. This paper briefly addresses itself to quite another question, which is to consider to what extent research can be expected to influence policy in the area of drug dependence. It would be beyond the scope of this paper to review all those instances in which the results of investigations have or have not had implications for decision making. The brief which will be taken is simply to enumerate some of the constraints which seem to affect the co-ordination of research and policy in this area.

Few would doubt the value to be gained from a more systematic application of the results of social science to the formulation and assessment of social policy, or question the fact that to some extent our continued pursuance of more and more research in the absence of any attempt to apply what is already known constitutes an extravagance of misplaced priorities. That a communication gap separates those whose profession it is to conduct

---

* Proceedings of the Second International Institute on the Prevention and Treatment of Drug Dependence, Baden, Austria, June 1971. International Council on Alcohol and Addictions.

research in the social sciences from those with responsibility for the decisions affecting such matters, is perhaps one of the greatest obstacles to the evolution of a planned society whose legislation is not dictated by political expedience but both anticipates its potential effects and attempts to monitor its actual effects. While to suggest that there is an automatic progression in the physical sciences linking theory, development and application is undoubtedly an oversimplification, the fact that the results of research in the social sciences rarely have market value means that this progression is even more tenuous. The fact that the abolition of the rum ration could have been advocated in 1834 for almost precisely the same reasons as were adduced in 1970 (Edwards and Jaffe, 1970) when eventually the ration was withdrawn, reveals something of the time scale affecting the application of research findings in this field. That in the United Kingdom we could have adopted a system of maintenance prescribing of heroin and methadone in 1968 and only in 1971 contemplated a controlled trial of the comparative efficacy of these two approaches provides a more contemporary example. Nevertheless there is evidence of an increasing concern for the utilisation of research (Social Science Research Council, 1969; Wootton, 1967; Watson, 1970; Cherns, 1967, 1968, 1969) and a dawning awareness of the essential wastefulness of a system of increasing public support for research which neither precludes duplication nor guarantees the application of results once discovered.

Part of the explanation of the detachment of research and policy making in this area undoubtedly lies in the complexity and subtlety of the relationship; part, however, resides in the different dispositions and training of the people concerned.

The research workers

Those engaged in research, usually academics, have traditionally seen their principal obligation to lie with their discipline. In pursuing research and scholarship they are motivated to contribute to the systematic body of knowledge making up their particular speciality. This affection has not usually included any attachment to the application of this knowledge, and indeed some researchers would dissociate themselves from any responsibility for the application of their research findings and assume instead a neutral or amoral attitude towards their discoveries. This view is expressed by one distinguished academic administrator in the following quotation: 'The social structure and purpose of the university accentuate the pressure toward purity. For the university's purpose is not to solve problems that are set for it outside a discipline. The university is not mission-orientated. Its purpose is to create and encourage the intellectual life *per se*. . . . In the universities it is improper

211

to ask the student, "What is the relevance of what you are doing to the rest of the world or even to the rest of science?" The acceptable question is, "What do your scientific peers, who view your work with the same intellectual prejudices as you, think of your work . . .?" ' (quoted in Cherns, 1970). Nor does the system of academic promotion demand that the researcher be able to show that his investigations have implications for the wider society. The research worker is not pressed therefore by professional affiliation or claims of personal advancement to publicise his findings beyond their presentation in some learned journal in a language comprehensible to his peers but frequently totally meaningless to those who might be thought to have an investment in their application.

There is also within the academic tradition the highly invested notion of academic freedom – a freedom which both ensures the immunity of the researcher against government and society's demands and allows him the right to investigate whatever problems he chooses. Given such autonomy the researcher is prone to react strongly to any suggestion that his research be directed or that his choice of research topic be decided in the light of a system of external priorities. While no one would doubt the benefits of this freedom it must at least be questioned whether one of its undesirable effects has not been the impotence of the academic, so that while he may undertake whatever research he chooses, his findings, whatever they are, can have no implication for the world outside the university. Having disdained any sense of public accountability the academic has forfeited any claim to a public audience.

The academic's prime commitment to his discipline also results in a tendency to construe specific issues as part of a more general process or perspective. Solving a particular problem is seen by the academic as only having value if it has implications for other problems and if his brief allows him to pursue these other implications. Those who administer policy and who have the responsibility for deciding between options are usually more empirical in their approach. They are concerned with the solution of a particular problem or a particular choice – they are less often interested in theoretical implications or in pursuing the solution of other hypothetical problems.

The policy makers

In contrast to those who pursue research, those Civil Servants and Ministers responsible for deciding questions of social policy are accountable to the public; indeed the whole fabric of democratic government rests on the premise of public accountability. Politicians are therefore not only concerned with what is right or true in the scientific sense but what is expedient or functional

212

in the political sense. In some instances these two systems of values will coincide; in others, however, they will be in conflict and politicians will react to their differing claims in different ways.

Nor does only political expedience affect decisions to implement policies; political dogma also plays a part. In some circumstances the particular dogma of the governing party can be expected to both dictate the approach made to a problem and to colour any assessment of its solution.

A system of parliamentary government which allows an opposition and thus the possibility of discontinuity in government also imposes a certain time scale on the decision-making process. Parties make promises which they must then enact or rescind within a prescribed period. Research cannot always be initiated and analysed with the same facility. Nor is it possible always to anticipate a particular piece of legislation and so evaluate its potential outcome; nor is there always the facility or even the willingness to evaluate legislation once it has been enacted. Superimposed on the time scale of governments is the even shorter tenure of ministers whose personality may in some instances at least be expected to influence decision making in the departments for which they are responsible.

In that political decisions are affected by a multitude of considerations additional to those affecting the conduct and outcome of research, the results of any investigation may be deemed expendable at the time of their eventual publication, whatever enthusiasm attended their initiation.

Further compounding these obstacles to relating research and policy is the tradition of anonymity and secrecy within the Civil Service. The confidentiality of some of the material affecting government policy decisions precludes making it available to outside researchers. The anonymity imposed on individuals by the Civil Service makes its constraints an unattractive career prospect for research workers.

The outcome of these differences has been on the one hand that much academic research is thought to be irrelevant in government circles, and on the other the view prevalent among academics that decisions taken by governments are often uninformed and compromised. Obviously neither of these assessments is wholly true nor should they be regarded as inevitable.

Common factors

In addition to those factors residing in the training or responsibilities of the two professions involved, there are common constraints affecting the rapprochement of research and policy in the area of drug dependence.

There is first and foremost the complexity of the problem. This complexity assumes a number of forms; it includes the undoubted multi-causal nature of the phenomenon – the fact that an explanation cast in exclusively pharmacological, personal or social terms is inadequate. It includes the unpredictability of the phenomenon – the fact that drug dependence has betrayed a bewildering variety of forms involving drugs of quite different pharmacological action; the abuse of some drugs and the disdain of others equally addictive. This unpredictability includes the uncertain outcome of any control or preventive measure undertaken. Drug education undertaken in some schools has been credited with heightening the interest of otherwise naive students. Proposals to reduce the use of prison sentences in the rehabilitation of drunkenness offenders by replacing sentences with fines merely resulted in the postponement of imprisonment when the majority of fines were not paid. Restrictive measures undertaken in one city, so reducing the availability of drugs, may succeed at the expense of causing drug users to migrate to other cities where such measures can be less easily implemented. It is probable that there can be no 'local' solution to the control of the drug problem in the same way as there can probably be no national solution without international implications.

In the face of this complexity the social sciences, and indeed all the sciences, have an inadequate conceptual framework and only amateurish machinery of assessment at their disposal. Research in this area still tends to be basically descriptive – it rarely sets out explicitly to test stated hypotheses. Its explanatory power is therefore low. It relies on verbal report and that from an audience of uncertain truthfulness and unreliable memory. It has not the benefit of an independent third party. Its conclusions are inevitably probablistic and even significant results are subject to equivocality. Its description of events is coloured by the rationalisations of the individual who has become dependent and the construction of those who have been observers of this process and possibly personally involved in it. Confronting the intricacies of the problem the social scientist has, to quote Marshall (1963), a 'relative shortage of apparatus which makes it difficult to provide schemes of analysis by which complicated problems are reduced to simple formulae'.

Finally, there is the difficulty of extrapolating the results of research investigations over time and place and even of repeating social experiments in the same context. Affected as they are by a whole collage of factors, programmes of prevention and treatment of drug dependence are rarely transferable as package deals. While the increase in the number of liquor outlets in Finland may have been associated with a significant increase in the consumption of alcohol, a similar liberalisation of the licensing laws in the United Kingdom need not have a similar effect, given the different degrees of urbanisation in the two countries, as only one example of their multitudinous differences. Nevertheless not to consider the implications of such liberalisation in other countries when contemplating it in the United Kingdom would seem to be the height of public irresponsibility.

Bridging the gap between research and policy will also however require that both researchers and those responsible for formulating policy make adjustments. It will demand of the researcher a greater recognition of the complexity of political decision making. While attuned to the complexity of his own discipline, the researcher often has a naive conception of the mechanisms of political decision. He may assume, for example, that because a certain decision is right or justified in the scientific sense, it is expedient. It needs to be recognised in addition that information, however complete, will be evaluated in terms of the policy makers' theories and values and that these, as much as inadequate information, will contribute to wrong decisions. The research worker also too often discounts the need to familiarise himself with the audience for his findings – he assumes that proof which is for him convincing is universally persuasive. In a sense one might claim that to demonstrate an association between lung cancer and cigarette smoking is irrelevant except that we also concern ourselves with ascertaining how those who smoke cigarettes may be aided in giving them up, if in fact they desire this.

The closer alignment of research and policy, if it is not to be delayed indefinitely, will also require a certain audacity of the researcher – a willingness to commit himself on the basis of incomplete evidence. For the researcher to claim that such decisions should not be taken reveals a naivety about the processes of government and a somewhat romantic conception of the proponents of policy. In all probability decisions must always be taken on the basis of incomplete data and that of the social researcher may on occasions be less incomplete than that of other more influential parties.

A rapprochement will also require that the academic forbear retreating into a pure/applied dichotomy which argues that the academic's only concern is with pure research. What is pure and what is applied research is at any one point of time a relative state of affairs, and probably tells us more about what efforts have been made to apply research than it does about the inherent characteristics of the research itself.

It is at least dubious whether the pure/applied distinction can be maintained at all in the social sciences. The difficulty of simulating the situations studied by the social sciences in contrived settings perhaps leaves no alternative but to study such phenomena in their natural surroundings with all the complexity that ensues. Boulding (1967) has commented that: 'By and large the social sciences have not been ambitious enough to want to study the socio sphere as a totality. They have been content with the kind of professional advancement which comes from the adequate processing of small pieces of information.

They have not had the larger vision of the study of the socio sphere as a totality'.

The choice confronting the social scientist has been depicted as that between studying insignificant questions with adequate methodology or countenancing significant questions with as yet inadequate methodology; to date, the former alternative would appear to be more often adopted.

Along with this need to assume a wider perspective, but inevitably seen by researchers as involving a loss of sovereignty, is the need for social research to be co-ordinated. There are many difficulties besetting any attempt to plan research or decide on areas of priority not least of which is the possibility that innovation will be retarded; equally, however, the pursuance of academic individualism is likely to result in needless redundancy. The United Kingdom Social Science Research Council in their 1969–70 Report (1970) attempted to steer a middle course between these two alternatives in that while discounting any attempt to devise a selective research strategy which would involve a policy of rejection, they expressed a preference for collective effort and advocate an attack on identified groups of problems.

There is, however, a more pressing need than the avoidance of unnecessary duplication recommending greater co-ordination in the social sciences. It can be argued that the nature of the phenomenon studied demands a multi-disciplinary approach and moreover a willingness to accommodate a degree of complexity which few individual researchers can countenance. In the absence of such co-ordination one can expect a proliferation of individually conceived studies fraught by many of the same methodological limitations. In so far as co-ordination exists in the present framework of research sponsorship it exists informally by virtue of the fact that the same people have membership on a number of grant-giving or advisory committees. What direction is lent research planning and what focusing on specific problems occurs, results from the informal influence members have in pressing certain needs and subsequently in advertising the availability of funds for the investigation of these needs. Less often will a grant-giving body formally declare its priorities.

Along with the avoidance of duplication and the achievement of greater economy and direction in research the closer alignment of research and policy will allow the test of hypotheses normally outside the province of the researcher. The very little positive evidence which exists pertaining to the efficacy of educative programmes reflects in large measure the fragmented application which has characterised most such programmes. That attempts to modify attitudes and behaviour have been attended by so little success is hardly surprising when it is considered that the vast majority of such efforts have amounted to the occasional and brief exposure of an audience to influences of dubious credibility in the face of a whole climate of contradictory influence. In the United Kingdom, for example, it was shown that the effect of a health education programme directed at schoolboy smoking was qualified in terms of whether the headmaster of the school concerned smoked or not.

One very considerable advantage of much closer co-operation between research workers and policy makers is that research might be mounted on a scale encompassing influences of an order which could be thought to provide a reasonable test of the hypothesis in question. While an increasing number of countries have implemented educative or preventive programmes little attempt has been made to assess their efficacy. While recognising the difficulties of attempting such evaluation, not the least of which is the time scale which must be entertained, it nevertheless needs to be recognised that it is essentially illogical to pursue further programmes in this area without evaluating the usefulness of existing programmes or anticipating the evaluation of projected programmes at the planning stage. The same could be said of changes in legislation affecting the availability of drugs. To date little advantage appears to have been taken systematically to examine the implications of legislative revision. Lacking evaluation, educative programmes and legal reform must otherwise be based on informed opinion and supported by impressionistic observation.

The same tolerance for ambiguity, if not downright contradictoriness, is evidenced in other contexts. In a recent Question Time in the British Houses of Parliament a member who protested it was ridiculous to identify drug taking with the permissive society was offered the following rebuff by the Minister responsible, 'I thought the words "permissive society" included that matter'. In the same Question Time a member concerned that 'outmoded restrictions on licensees be got rid of ', the effect of which would be to increase the availability of alcohol, and who wanted the whole business of licensing laws reviewed, was promised by the same Minister that such a review would take place 'as speedily as possible' (Edwards, 1971).

The better co-ordination of research and legislation in this area in addition to contributing to more rational national policy, would also allow advantage to be taken of the various 'natural experiments' which occur on an international scale. It is obviously impossible for the research worker to contrive all those circumstances which would provide a test of his hypotheses – it may indeed be unethical for him to presume this – nevertheless there occur a number of interesting natural experiments of a similar nature which are not always investigated. The prolonged and chronic use of cannabis in some of the North African countries is one such example as is the proliferation of rehabilitation facilities in the United States.

In addition to concerning himself with what have been identified as significant problems, that is, in this context problems having policy implications, the audacity required of the social science researcher will demand that he give much more attention to those processes affecting the acceptance of facts. Cherns (1968) has observed that, 'I have not been able to trace in practice one example of a study carried out in a university or research institute or anywhere else which resulted in direct application except where the researcher had become involved in following through his studies into application'. This involvement is in marked contrast to the researcher's traditional disinterest which has been achieved by equating the concepts of value and science. For a researcher to claim no responsibility for his discoveries is to some extent irresponsible; it assumes that those who are responsible for its application are somehow better informed of its implications. While researchers may retort that at least those who are responsible are accountable to the public, what has been argued here would recommend that social scientists should be equally accountable not only in their choice of problems for investigation but in explaining the implications of their findings. It is fallacious to assume that there are informed and impartial 'middle men' whose function it is to interpret the social sciences to those responsible for implementing social policy — lacking such honest brokers social scientists must at least ask whether they are not themselves the best equipped to undertake this function.

To concentrate on the need for social scientists to make certain adjustments may be seen as implying that only they are responsible for the present detachment of research and policy. Similar adjustments will also be required of the administrator if he is to accept Wootton's (1967) 'workable model of the future', which envisages advice being given on policy by those who are 'competent to use and to interpret the results of modern research techniques and who are serviced by staffs equipped to assist them in this task'. At least some of the secrecy affecting certain issues of public importance needs to be reduced if adequate and independent information is to be obtained on the implications of the several options possible. Ministers and those who advise them must likewise agree to anticipate certain decisions if research findings are to contribute to the decision-making process. Similarly when legislation has been introduced, facilities must be found for monitoring its effect or at least some aspects of its effect, if more than political persuasion is to affect the formation of public policy. There may be grounds in some instances for introducing legislation on an experimental basis where a deliberate attempt is made to assess the outcome and where amendments are made in the light of these findings. While such a self-correcting process exists at present its course is probably more irrational and cumbersome than would result if an assessment of outcome was an integral part of the legislation when introduced.

One of the difficulties affecting the assessment of social legislation is of course predicting outcome and thus identifying the relevant variables to measure. The end product of such legislation is likely to be elusive and only tenuously and belatedly related to its manipulations. In the same way the actual impact of research on policy is a matter of considerable subtlety. While in the United Kingdom the so-called Wootton Report was rejected by the then Home Secretary, but despite the fact that following its publication there has been no revision of the penalties associated with cannabis offences, in reality the practice of the courts has gradually approximated to the recommendations of the report.

There should also be more communication between administrators and researchers. At present there exist few forums where an increasing acquaintance with each others' problems and points of view is engendered.

Related to this need for more communication between social scientists and administrators is the need for both to be implicated in the research undertaken. Both should be persuaded that the appropriate questions are being asked and both committed to an examination of their conclusions. While the volume and expense of research commissioned by government departments has increased enormously in recent years (Armstrong, 1969), few would claim that adequate return has been achieved from the investment. Orlans (1968) concluded after a mammoth review of government-sponsored social research in the United States that 'not one of the government agencies providing money for social research was able to offer a true evaluation of the use it had made of the research it had sponsored'. A greater commitment to examine the utilisation of research may result if sponsoring agencies required some consideration of the possible implications of the results in the initial proposal and, in appropriate circumstances, if they themselves agreed to finance the 'development' stage of the investigation.

Perhaps when social scientists own an increasing obligation to the society which supports them and governments have a greater willingness to allow their decisions to be informed by social research, the potential significance of the social sciences in the ordering of man's social environment will be realised, and the facility man has acquired for advancing his material welfare will be matched by a greater capacity to solve those problems concerning his relationship with his fellow men.

33   Listening to 99*

ALAN OGBORNE

Summary

A social scientist sets out some of the usual charges which are today levelled at the irrelevance of research by those who are concerned with social action and making the world a better place. He suggests that these charges should be taken seriously and proceeds to an examination of the main headings. The complex and not necessarily benign influence of the research process on the subject who is actually being studied is in particular given note.

Some people don't believe in social research. They think it's a waste of time, energy and money. They accuse researchers of living in ivory towers, being overpaid, of lacking commitment and of being pawns in the political game of sustaining the *status quo*. We are further said to be unfeeling, unconcerned with suffering, interested only in what other researchers think about us and of writing reports for those equally detached from the real world. We are charged with finding out at enormous cost what everybody knows anyhow and of expressing ourselves in terms which serve merely to mask the fact that our views are no more profound than those of the average layman.

Heretics draw near. You will find your charges taken seriously. Doubters are found even among the ranks of the faithful, but do not use them as a stick to beat us, rather make some constructive contribution to a continuing debate. What is the proper role of research in society's response to social problems?

Social scientists are very good at asking questions, most of which are as yet unanswered and not a few are probably unanswerable. As men and women, then, they must master the art of doubt. As scientists they seek information which could invalidate their views on the world and which may reflect back on the very nature of their discipline. As social beings they must call themselves into question since they are part of that which is in doubt. As theorists they must be able to account for themselves (or deny their social nature) and as practitioners they must develop the capacity to assess their personal contribution to the dynamics of research situations. For those engaged in the study of social problems such an art must be practised in the

---

* A paper written specially for this volume.

context of doubts as to the definition of that which is studied, doubts as to the need for study and the thought that one's labours will serve no useful purpose.

To study or to act? Not *the* question but one often asked. Can social problems be solved by more research? Could it even be, as some of our harshest critics have proclaimed, that the setting up of research is a way of avoiding action? Aren't social problems after all 'symptoms' of the society in which we live; we don't need research to tell us that we have to act. Researchers just sit on the fence, indulging in the luxury of non-commitment, distracting attention from the *real* causes of social problems and those in whose interests the *status quo* is organised. To those who level such charges I would say that if their claims are valid the good researcher will not hesitate to join their chorus of protest and his research, if well planned and thought out, can do no harm to honest causes. There are many forces which bring about change; perhaps good research could be given more attention.

Yet are we concerned with action? Isn't research something to do with being 'scientific', 'objective', with being committed only to the non-commitment of the tentative hypothesis and the testable (and thus rejectable) theory? Aren't all those chi-squares and rotated factors, signs of our scientism; and thus (by erroneous implication) indicative of our lack of concern for people?

There are many types of researchers. Some are dedicated to the idea of a 'scientific' social science, partly as an academic exercise but also because they believe in the possibility of a rational society; a society which makes decisions on the basis of 'where it's at' and not because of vested interests. There are those who are occupied with the refinement of the tools of their trade, with developing better interviewing techniques, more reliable attitude scales, more refined statistical analysis. Others are theoreticians and while equally concerned with the quality of data they are devoted to the development and refinement of theoretical systems, again partly as an academic exercise though often with a direct concern for social action since the basic assumptions of social policies are of theoretical interest.

Then there are those who feel that research ideas, techniques and the research 'mentality' can be employed directly in the alleviation of suffering, sometimes by working with individuals, more often through contacts with social workers or with those responsible for major policy decisions. This latter group have the problem of having to employ ill-developed research techniques and sometimes the rescarcher–practitioner partnership gives rise to conflicts.

But researchers are not easy creatures to categorise nor are they unamenable to discussion as to what research is all about. Most of them occasionally doubt the value of their work and odd cries of 'what is it all about?' can be heard echoing along the corridors. In such a phase, the researcher, like millions of others, does his job and goes home.

Yet isn't research a form of action anyhow? We do meet people, and however 'scientific' we may try to be during encounters we must as human beings have some effect on them. Some sociologists have defined social problems in terms of social response. Problem areas are those aspects of society towards which actions are directed. Research is part of a social response. What impact does it have on the problems to which it is addressed?

Even (or especially?) the most hard-headed of the 'scientific' scientists recognise that people affect each other. (Some have had to do studies to show that this is the case but that's another story!)

Social research is not carried out by one group of rational, self-directed, disinterested people on inert substances or non-rational, responsive beings controlled by forces from which the researchers are immune. Rather it involves the meeting of two or more rational/non-rational, creative/responsive, sane/crazy, human beings who must together negotiate the definition of the research situation. The 'unco-operative' subjects (respondents, interviewees), those coded 99 or rated as 'unreliable', are not beyond research though they tend to mess up one's research design and restrict the representativeness of one's sample. Rather they are people who don't share the researcher's definition of reality, they do not know or they won't abide by the ground rules of the game. Their refusal or inability to play will itself form the basis of the good researcher's attention, though we are sometimes guilty of merely recording 'not known', lamenting the complexities of social life and neglecting the social nature of social research. If we tempered our scientism with a little more sensitivity we might learn a deal more about whom we claim to study and be forced to look more carefully at some of our boasts of objectivity.

Apart from influencing how they behave towards us, what else do we do to those whom we deliberately seek out for interviews? Probably not very much in view of the comparative shortness of most research contacts. But are we not sometimes guilty of collusion? The successful interview is after all the one in which subjects play our game, the one in which we get confirmed in our chosen roles. Don't we by the same token agree to confirm (collude?) with our subjects' sense of self? By what right do we faithfully record hard-luck stories or tales of how clever it is to get stoned or drunk? Why should we passively sit back and listen to the sacred attitudes of people whom any fool can tell are talking nonsense? And what of those with real problems and a genuine need for help, the ones who agree to be seen because they want someone to talk to about their troubles? Research can seem horribly shallow when all you have to offer is a series of 'yes'/'no' questions about doing this, going there, using that, how much?, how often?, when did you first start?, and so on.

222

There are many unresolved problems. Being the objects of research may well affect some people in undesirable ways. We may confirm their self-delusions, their commitment to deviance, or just upset them because we have asked about things which have great emotional significance. Even questions about age, sex and social class can cause difficulties to people who don't know their age, are uncertain of their gender and who never knew their parents.

Ultimately our lack of sustained concern with the particular reflects our commitment to the importance of the general. One unhappy addict does not invalidate a clinic system. Sixty per cent unhappy from a well chosen sample says far more. Likewise one 'cured' alcoholic from a rehabilitation hostel does not prove that the treatment works. He must stand alongside those who have relapsed, those who stopped drinking unaided and those helped by other agencies. Good evaluation research demands a rigorous experimental design. But how cold we must sound to the dedicated social worker whose 'failures', even more than his successes, have demanded more emotional tax than most researchers could ever pay.

One day we might hear a social scientist shout 'eureka!' It's unlikely, but there may be facts and laws of social life yet to be 'discovered'. Perhaps a wandering tribe of alcoholics with previously undreamed of drinking patterns. Perhaps a variable which explains over 60 per cent of the variation of drug addicts' abstinence. Perhaps, but unlikely. Most social science findings (we are not prone to say discoveries) are not altogether surprising. Somebody, somewhere, probably knew or suspected them all along, though without the precision which research can bring.

But why do research? Opinions vary and relate to one's optimism, or otherwise, that any attention will be paid to one's work. Some researchers even claim to be unconcerned with social action. The researcher—reformer is, they say, neither a good researcher (since his commitment precludes neutrality), nor a good action man (since his pretence at neutrality probably masks his lack of real commitment). Others believe that good data lends strength to good causes. Facts and figures did after all help to bring home the horrors of slavery, though presumably everybody knew that some slaves died in the ships, and those in touch could have made a pretty good guess at how many. Surveys on the poverty of the aged or the plight of the homeless help to complete a picture whose general shape is well known, but whose full horror needs the clarity of well collected data. Everybody knows that a lot of prisoners have drinking problems and that some alcoholics get sent down regularly, but armed with good data one can feel more confident in attacking an inhuman, unproductive system.

What of explanation? Can research help us to understand the world? I once tried to explain to an intelligent secretary why it was that a Slough mini-cab driver with a fast car didn't overtake a slower cab on his way back to the rank. I mustered all I knew of group dynamics, theories of primal hoards, the economics of cab driving, existential psychology, and proudly concluded my thesis with some remark about the value of social science to the understanding of human behaviour. When she replied that he didn't overtake because he didn't want his colleagues to disapprove of him for jumping the queue, I confessed to being somewhat deflated. It's much the same with all those 'intelligent laymen' who tell me that they think that people take drugs because they are influenced by their friends or that they are curious, or that they are unhappy and are trying to escape from their problems, etc. After years of research can we really say anything which, when you get right down to it, is any more profound or original? The trouble with being a social scientist is that everyone has his own views on the whys and wherefores of human behaviour, and it is not uncommon (in fact it's pretty well always the case) that their views are remarkably like those found in your actual learned journals – suitably translated into jargon of course. Personally, I'd be suspicious of social science if it got too far removed from common sense. Perhaps one of our roles is to refine common sense, to systematise it ... to mobilise it? We do after all have the privilege of time to think about problems in detail.

Despite all doubts, research continues. Questionnaires get punched, computers, when they don't eat your cards or blow up, produce print-outs, reports are written and new publications appear. By this time those involved may be so fed up that they are happy to move on to further projects. But the report on the desk raises the questions with which one began. Why do this study? Who is it for? What action does it suggest? Who can take such action? Will they?

Members of the Addiction Research Unit are concerned about the use of research. Many have direct involvements with action projects and others move round the corridors of power doing their best to bring research to the attention of the right people. Perhaps current practising researchers should see movement towards a direct involvement with policy-making as a worthwhile career. The research mind with its capacity for entertaining and synthesising different ways of looking at things and its respect for data, should be of value in decision making. The good researcher, because he moves in a variety of circles, will have perspectives on the world which are denied to others. If he is researching into dependency he should know a great deal about what it's like to be a drug addict or an alcoholic. He will know about the courts, the prisons, social workers, probation officers, voluntary agencies, professional workers. His knowledge of decision making may be limited but having familiarised himself with the multitude of variables which are important in a particular problem area, the mature researcher may with due modesty be able to make a positive contribution to social policy making.

But there are those who thrive on the research business itself; whose commitment to the improvement of their disciplines takes precedence over their wish to change the world. Perhaps the two are forever intimately related. Karl Marx felt that his followers should be more concerned to change the world than to understand it. But as a good social scientist he recognised the relationship between theory, action, and data.

34   Statistics as they turn out*

PETER NICHOLLS

Summary

A statistician discusses the relevance of conventional statistical trains to the demands made of him on joining a research unit. The role of the statistician in such a setting is mixed. He must be able to meet simple service needs and act as consultant who advises on more complex problems of design and analysis. His role is also in many ways that of continued educator.

The great majority of postgraduate courses in statistics in this country aim at presenting to the student a wide range of statistical theories and methods of analysis. Much emphasis is put on the mathematical basis of the statistics concerned – topics such as statistical inference, stochastic processes, multivariate analysis, computer programming and analysis of variance – in the expectation that those students who graduate will be able to work in any field which presents itself, be it economics, medicine, agriculture, operational research or some other. Very few courses are available which aim to train statisticians for specific fields of work, though their number has recently increased. Such specialised courses, while still presenting a broad education in statistics, also concentrate on statistical applications in their chosen field and therefore are of much more practical use to the student.

Coming straight from a postgraduate course of the more traditional type I viewed the statistician's job as that of a 'problem solver'. The statistician would supply advice in designing experiments or projects, and similarly help-out at the analysis stage. Should something go wrong, then it would be up to him to recover the situation in the best way possible. In terms of how I would spend my time working at the Addiction Research Unit my chief task would be to provide this sort of statistical service to a group of chiefly medical personnel engaged in various forms of treatment trials and other research. A number of forms of statistical analysis would no doubt prove useful, particularly multivariate analysis and the analysis of variance.

Julian Peto and I joined company in the Addiction Research Unit in October 1970. Our rather small shared room overlooking the tennis court

---

* A paper written specially for this volume.

gave us a pleasant view of the hospital and Institute, and thanks to the willingness of our new colleagues to come along and talk statistics it was not long before we were able to gain an overall impression of the status of the research that was going on within the Unit. The number of incomplete projects was in the region of 20, of which some half dozen were needing analysis and the remainder were at the data collection stage. There was no immediate prospect of working on new projects, since at that time none was being planned. Some backlog of work had built up over the previous two or three years as a result of poor computing facilities; the considerable number of boxes of cards cluttering our room bore eminent testimony to this. By somewhat arbitrary means we divided the various jobs between ourselves and so began our work.

During the time I spent at the Addiction Unit I was involved in the work for a large proportion of the projects but the great majority of my time was spent on three particular projects, each at an advanced stage of completion. The research had been planned up to five years previously and in each case the collection of data had been continuing for some two or more years. Given this situation, it was not surprising that research workers in the Unit were more interested in what I as a statistician had to say about analysis of data rather than collection of data. But analysis of data must inevitably depend on correct methods being used as the data is collected and there were occasions when errors had been made at the planning stage, certain sets of data being as a result of only limited value. In the circumstances it was necessary to make the best use possible of such data, but at the same time to note that an important role for the statistician was to educate researchers in the ways of designing and planning their work so that they are in fact able to test their hypotheses at the end of the day. Those who embark on their work without any prior statistical advice as regards its design meet with difficulties at a later stage.

Having overcome certain design problems and decided on a certain form of analysis for the data in hand, the temptation is always very strong to set off for the calculating machine or computer and 'get some answers'. Statisticians as well as other research workers often suffer from this complaint. It soon became clear however that such action was jumping the gun and that data had to be looked at very carefully and thoroughly checked before detailed analysis could begin. A number of things govern the reliability of data punched on a computer data card and each of these has to be checked. Is the layout of the questionnaire/coding schedule easy to follow? Are the codes well defined and mutually exclusive? How are missing values coded? How is the data punched on to the data cards? Is the punching accurate? That each of these things is checked is vital to the analysis of a set of data and it is very important that this data checking stage should not be omitted. During my time at the Unit I wrote a series of instructions for the design of questionnaires and included in these details of card punching facilities and a number of purpose-written computer programmes which would produce frequency counts for a large number of variables together with various summary statistics. These programmes required a minimum of computer knowhow and research workers were on occasions able to set up and run the jobs for themselves. The frequency counts programme produced a detailed summary of the data punched and having checked this data and corrected any mistakes, it is then possible to continue with confidence to further analysis.

The majority of projects in the Addiction Unit have social scientists in a key role and the approach to the work is therefore somewhat different from that in medical research generally, and indeed from what I had expected. Projects which seek to find definitions for a problem or to trace its natural history, retrospectively or prospectively, must necessarily involve the collection of large amounts of data, especially so when the research is interdisciplinary and social workers, psychologists, psychiatrists and sociologists are all involved. Whether dealing with dependence on alcohol or tobacco or any kind of drug, all agree that the problem is multi-dimensional and that there is no simple answer. The danger at this point is to assume that a difficult problem can be solved by making use of an advanced form of statistical analysis, such as multivariate analysis. There are occasions when some form of multivariate analysis will be ideal for a given set of data but in most cases the underlying distributional and theoretical requirements render it inapplicable. My view is that it is a mistake to make wide use of such forms of analysis, especially in a situation where the methods are not fully understood. Given the limited statistical knowledge of those involved in the research much more straightforward techniques proved equally useful and far easier to interpret, cross tabulation techniques especially so. On the occasions when a form of multivariate analysis was used it was necessary to make sure that the research worker concerned was aware of the assumptions he was making about his data and was able to interpret the results correctly.

In conclusion my role in the Addiction Unit can perhaps best be summed up by saying that I sought to provide statistical advice and aid whenever needed at whatever stage of a project. It was a service role in that I was, along with Julian Peto, responsible for almost all the analysis of a large number of projects, but there was also a very important education role, which for myself involved giving advice on the principles involved in the design of projects, the preparation of data for analysis and the applications of various forms of statistical analysis.

35   Exploring the role of the information scientist*

MAXINE MacCAFFERTY

Summary

An information scientist's potential contribution to the work of a multi-disciplinary research team is explored. The continuing problem is how most effectively to build and maintain the working liaison between the information specialist and the research team: research workers have to learn how best to use the resources of this rather new speciality.

The Addiction Research Unit's library arose from the need to store material that had been collected over the years by individual researchers. Eventually, the material was organised to facilitate storage and retrieval of information, and consisted principally of a reprint collection and a few books and journals. As the Unit staff and research projects grew in number, it became necessary to make the library a more powerful source of assistance rather than just a repository.

The reprint collection is now expanding at a much faster rate, covering literature in the addictions field generally, as well as the subject areas of the research projects in particular. Books and specialised periodicals are being acquired with the same view in mind. The classification system in use at present, for the reprints only, will soon be inadequate, and a more flexible system will have to be introduced. What form it will take has yet to be decided.

The article reprints once received are exhaustively indexed. This means that precision of the subject matter sought is lowered, as many papers might not be solely concerned with all the keywords used, but recall is high thus ensuring that fringe material is usually retrieved. Precision is the required relevancy of the retrieved material. High precision indicates that few articles will be irrelevant (these would be called false drops), but depending on the efficacy of the retrieval system used, it might well mean that some such articles will remain undetected, and therefore be lost to the potential user. On the other hand, when precision is lowered, many papers will be retrieved which might cover the needed information only peripherally, or as a special

---

* A paper specially written for this volume.

aspect of some other major subject. This total quantity of retrieved papers is termed recall, and thus it can be seen that recall is high when precision is low, and vice versa.

For many reasons, there is a vast amount of material which the Unit library could not consider purchasing. The Institute of Psychiatry library and its inter-library loan services cater for these needs. Another facility is MEDLARS, the Medical Literature Analysis and Retrieval System, a computerised storage and retrieval system serving the medical field, to which a researcher may send various kinds of profiles of his needs. The Institute Library also holds the entire collection of abstract cards produced by the Rutgers Center of Alcohol Studies. The drug field can be surveyed by means of the exhaustive collection at the Institute for the Study of Drug Dependence elsewhere in London.

The Unit library produces a monthly bulletin of all material acquired. It is divided into broad subject categories, to enable rapid scanning of a particular field of interest. At present, it is not feasible to subdivide these categories into more specialised sections, but when the volume of material should cause difficulties, then subdivision would become appropriate. A reprint collection of all publications produced by the Unit staff is also kept. These reprints are available on request.

The information scientist is aware of the contents of all meetings, thus possibly gaining a background of research in formulation prior to any enquiry which might be forthcoming. Contacts with centres in our own field, both here and overseas, have been and are being made constantly.

Knowing the researchers and their research work assists one to know what kind of information is expected, and plans can be made accordingly to provide it.

There are two practical problems involving how best to ensure the researchers are aware of the latest papers in their sphere of interest. First, it is difficult to survey all the current work throughout the world. Secondly, in an interdisciplinary field, work in several areas of knowledge may be relevant, and it is virtually impossible to follow developments in all of them.

Scanning journals, though the most effective method of surveying written material, is just too time-consuming. Current awareness services must be used, giving one a great advantage where time is limited, and ensuring the majority of relevant literature is discovered. Only a small proportion of the total volume published will be missed.

Researchers need methods and systems which enable them to be familiar with current progress and the state of the art. They are facilitated by indexing and abstracting journals, and one's own stored information: the library. Information gathering can become an obsession, so any library collection should reflect a policy derived from the linkage between researchers' needs and the subject area.

The drug dependency field is truly interdisciplinary: for example, psychology, psychiatry, sociology, medicine, pharmacology. It is not just multi-disciplinary, for the various sciences overlap, and discoveries in any one of them can seriously affect progress in another. The researchers may not work in the isolation of their own discipline, so their information and all resources must be pooled. The information unit is the information pool.

The function of such a unit is twofold. First, it must act as a filter to select relevant material from the world's total information output. The sensitivity of the filter depends on the intercommunication between the information scientist and the researchers, both individually and as a team. There should be a useful degree of involvement with each other's work. The information worker should attempt to be an integral part of every research team, to know what research is going on, to know in what way new research proposals are being planned; in essence to know how every researcher thinks and conducts his art of investigation. It is not the information worker's purpose to become a subject specialist, but more to understand and adapt to the application of thought behind all scientific endeavour and to help fulfil that direction.

The exchange of information between people should not depend solely on the published word if it is to be a dynamic process. Personal communication is essential to enhance the spread of ideas.

The researcher integrates his individual thinking with that of his team. He probes his determined resources to see how his ideas might best be developed. Discussions should already be taking place with the information scientist. Thus, the second function of the information unit is recognised. It acts as a resource from which the researcher may draw, especially when he has a definite information need, but also in the preliminary stages when that need is itself being formulated. This is the occasion when questions are considered, such as these: how much information is needed; what is needed, by the individual, and by the team; how will it be provided? Derived from these practical considerations, are theoretical questions for the information worker: can the methods and systems available substitute for the well-read researcher; what are the special problems in drug dependency literature; how best can the researcher use those systems; what must be the particular role and responsibility of the information scientist?

This communication between researcher and information worker is often more difficult to obtain than the researcher's required information. Admittedly in the case of the Addiction Research Unit, the staff were not expecting to have an information scientist in their midst and indeed they were unaware that such a person could exist. But get one they did, and it is a

231

constant day-to-day effort to encourage them to communicate their research thinking and intentions, and their information needs. This situation is sadly common all over the world, and although the fundamental concepts and activities of information science have been well off the ground since intelligence operations during World War II, it has only recently become a recognised professional discipline. Educating researchers to maximise the usefulness of all their information sources, including their information worker, is but another aspect of the information scientist's role.

In the final analysis, only the researcher can determine the degree of usefulness of a certain paper. In this sense, there is no substitute for wide reading, and for this reason it is best for the information worker to err on the side of over-supply, with consideration of fringe subjects which might well cast fresh light and new thought on to the original ideas and plans.

36 The grass roots and the ivory tower: a personal view*

TIMOTHY COOK

Summary

The relationship between compassion and science sets problems. The relevance of the research which goes on in the addictions to human realities can seem remote to the social worker who witnesses the daily suffering. The need is for constructive dialogue rather than further polarisation of positions. Some possible questions for the agenda of that dialogue are considered.

The alcoholic gazes bleakly but rather admiringly at the rows of research reports and the volumes of the *Quarterly Journal of Studies on Alcohol* which rest in unordered piles just behind the doctor's head. The titles from time to time swim into focus and the volumes look impressive and the doctor seems even more learned than before. The alcoholic ventures a question, just forestalling the psychiatric probe that was about to come his way. 'Doctor, have you read all those books?' he asks. 'Why, yes', is the reply, 'in fact', he adds in a moment of unguarded immodesty, 'I wrote a few articles myself'. 'Do you find they've helped you understand the likes of me any better? I mean is all that research going to solve my problem?' 'Well, it's not quite as simple as that,' replies the doctor, 'research isn't always meant to help people you know. It is to increase knowledge and understanding, to pose questions, to widen horizons, to take intellectual risks – I suppose it might help you, or more likely your children, if they take to drink'. The alcoholic by now is bemused and rather wishing he hadn't started this conversation. He watches the titles go out of focus and eventually he leaves the room knowing that his doctor has written some learned papers but not sure whether he, the alcoholic, understands anything more than that.

'Grossly unfair', is probably how most research workers would react to the above scenario. Research does not after all set out to help people in the same way as social workers. It is too easy to polarise the division between research and social work in this way. Not only is it too easy, it is a disservice to both disciplines. The research worker will insist that we are all keen to assist our

---

* A paper written specially for this volume.

fellow man, only some choose to do it by one method and others by another. In any case research is not all that easy, you know! Readers of C. P. Snow are of course aware of the strange stresses of the academic life. But nonetheless, polarisation or not, my own experience is that it is rare for social workers and research workers really to meet in open dialogue, and when they do come together the issues rapidly become polarised and almost grotesque; human concern versus raw data; involvement versus detachment; individuals versus statistics; martyrs versus publication-hungry careerists; total availability to client versus office hours mentality; down to earth versus unreal and remote; human beings versus monster, or is it monsters versus human beings? But just what is the reality? How far do social workers really make use of research and how far are they encouraged to do so? How far does research even attempt to inform social work? Can we make some guesses at the truth within the fable of the grass roots and the ivory tower?

The first thing to note is that the problem is by no means new. In the last century Arnold Toynbee said that 'to make benevolence scientific is the great problem of the present age'. Since then, McDonald (1960) has said that 'the profession of social work has evolved to make scientific the organised benevolence of the community, using established fact and theory in its service, without reducing the practitioner to the status of a routine clinician, or divorcing from benevolence the element of compassion'. There is then some evidence to suggest that social work has sought to move away from anecdotal evidence of success and efficacy, to move away from the tendency to extrapolate from one soul searing case to a new total theory. In other parallel spheres, such as education, there have been some fine recent accounts of the judicious combination of science and compassion (e.g., Halsey, 1972). Nonetheless, social work can still be criticised (Wootton 1959) for a rather loose use of language and concept in trying to bolster up its desire for a new professional status. It would perhaps be honest to admit that some areas of social work still remain elusive for the researcher, and the tools of social science are simply not subtle enough to unravel all the human tangles that social work can present. Yet, because this is true of some areas, it should not be used to allow the social worker totally to dismiss research endeavours in the social work field. I personally always find it rather despairing, as I am sure researchers do, to hear social workers saying, 'Oh well, you can prove anything with statistics' and then proceeding to carry on in the same old ineffective way. Research, on the other hand, should not claim more than it can usefully do. For example, criminological predictions seem to me an example of a science trying to run before it can really walk. Whatever position we take up, I am sure most of us would agree that we have at least made some progress since the good Miss Theis (quote in McDonald, 1960) who in the

234

1920s in a follow up study of foster children took 'orderly prudence and good sense' as two of her criteria of adjustment. The practitioners need to pay attention to the research workers – where would we be without Bowlby? – we need to recognise that it is ultimately in the service of the client whom we profess to serve that attempts at evaluation of our work should be undertaken. Perhaps we need to accept, above all, that down in the grass roots there are some pretty murky swamps.

I personally, however, am much more concerned about the other side of the relationship, that is, how research workers view the practitioners, be they social workers or clinicians. It is only too easy of course for the outsider to poke fun at research – the rats racing around boxes, the mice being injected with vodka, pages of seemingly incomprehensible matrices, correlations, grids and graphs. John Osborne in *Look Back in Anger* ridiculed the recherché literary critics who debated in the columns of *The Times* whether Milton wore braces or not. Some research is clearly of that order, while other research is essential to the development of services for people with problems; social psychiatry would be a good example of the latter (Wing, 1973).

Within the field of addiction, however, I am not sure that addiction research units have ever seriously entered into a sane form of dialogue with the workers in the addiction field. There are questions that need to be debated between the two sides. If the research workers are not willing to consider these questions, then at least they should state why they do not regard them as relevant. I am myself responsible for a hostel for alcoholics being researched by two members of an addiction research unit. The research is important and yet some statements that are made and some of the preliminary findings I find incomprehensible, as I am sure the residents in the hostel do too. Is that an important fact or not? I believe it to be a crucial question for it raises just the problem of whom the research is for. The amount of research that is being conducted into alcoholism is phenomenal. It is, however, rarely read by field workers. Far too often, almost always indeed, the research seems to be written for other research workers to read and to comment upon and that in turn to be commented upon (e.g., Robinson, 1972, and comments). It is published in journals invariably inaccessible to most social workers, and even where obtainable is too frequently unintelligible. It seems to be published where it will have the most prestige and be seen by the greatest number of research colleagues. This is obviously fine for the career of the individual research worker, but at the same time unless some serious attempt is made consistently to communicate the findings of alcoholism research to other groups of workers, then the volumes of research will gather dust and become more sterile year by year.

Now I am not naive enough to believe that research will tell me how to deal with a particularly difficult drunk on a Monday morning, but I am optimistic enough to feel that if a more serious effort was made to relate alcoholism research to the problems of the practitioner and indeed, the problems of the client himself, then we should come to understand more about the whole phenomenon of alcoholism. There has been some excellent research done on the issue of motivation in alcoholics, the possibilities of social drinking amongst alcoholics, the value of the criteria of abstinence and other similar areas, absolutely germane to the work of any serious social worker dealing with an addict. The fact remains, however, that unless one has the good fortune to be in some chance contact with an addiction research unit, and to be on speaking terms with the workers in that unit, your life will pass by and your work continue without your being aware at all of the content of this kind of research.

Another question that really needs to be asked is why research one aspect as opposed to another? Research workers on the whole seem to talk with each other and plan their research with each other, rarely calling in the outside social workers. The social worker rarely has time to conduct serious research on his own, but nonetheless if he is a thinking and sensitive person, invariably faces a number of crucial questions during the course of any one week or any one month dealing with alcoholics. Many of these questions he might well like to have researched. But rarely is the opportunity given for these questions or these ideas to be discussed in a forum with people skilled in the art of research. The result too often seems to be that yet more papers and more journals are produced which take the whole subject matter further and further away from the realities facing the alcoholic and the helper. It is of course appreciated that in all research units there must be a degree of risk capital – the exploring of seemingly way out prospects, the willingness to pursue the uncertain. But not all research can or should be of this nature. My own particular interest is the field of homeless alcoholics, and questions which seem to me eminently researchable but which have remained unresearched (as far as I can tell) are why do some homeless alcoholics repeatedly get arrested for drunkenness and others rarely at all, why do some beg and steal and others not, how and why do some men become part of drinking gangs and others not? These are detailed investigations but not more detailed than studying ten or twenty mice, white or brown. Most social workers will probably feel that the dividends which would come from this kind of research are possibly greater than discovering whether most alcoholics shake on the third or the fourth day after they have stopped drinking. I am not arguing for social workers dictating the policy of an addiction research unit, but I am saying that unless there is a greater willingness on the part of research units to involve and invoke the ideas and experience of the social workers, then a

236

disservice is being done both to research and to the subject of the research.

A fourth question I would like to have debated is why research workers are so reluctant to make use of all the raw data that is literally lying at their feet, even though some of the data may be deficient in respects that make it difficult to fit into some rigorous ideal research design (Shyne, 1960; Mayer and Tims, 1970). In London, for example, there are probation offices and hostels for alcoholics that have been working in the field for ten or more years. There are filing cabinets literally bulging with files on alcoholics. Surely it would be worth knowing just what has happened to these alcoholics in the ten years, say, since they left the hostel. Such information could surely tell us a great deal of the pattern of movement of certain groups of alcoholics. I appreciate that this kind of research is perhaps rather tedious and less glamorous than some other kinds. Nonetheless one day it will surely have to be done. What I am asking is that debate about how and when it should be done should be started now.

Finally, I would like to say that it still strikes me as extraordinary that in an area of London where there is a proliferation of alcoholic agencies – indeed one journal was moved to comment that if you have to be an alcoholic then the best place to be is Camberwell – and also an Addiction Research Unit, that despite the proximity of these two groups of facilities there is only *ad hoc* communication between them. That state of affairs has not happened simply by chance. There are built in resistances on both sides. One side doesn't like statistics, the other side doesn't like the account of individual cases. Neither side should allow it to continue. Research policies and social work policies should be worked out together. If a start could be made in this kind of direction, then I believe that in a subsequent edition of this book somebody could continue the fable of the grass roots and the ivory tower. Hopefully the fable would not end with the ivory tower becoming so big and so large that it could no longer see the grass roots. Nor indeed would it end with the grass roots growing and growing and overwhelming and suffocating the ivory tower. No, the fable could surely have an ending which goes something like 'and they lived happily ever after'.

37 Appraisal

In that well worn phrase these five papers raise more questions than they answer. The questions go under two broad headings. There are first those issues related to how a complex research unit best orders its own internal life, and here the matters raised by a statistician and by an information scientist are only examples of the more general organisational problems of the modern research life. Secondly there are a host of questions bearing on the external relations of a research unit.

Some might argue that the balance of this book reflects indeed the very imbalance of which critics of the research world complain. They would say that there is too much research being churned out by the research industry, with too little consideration as to whether the goods are those the shopper actually needs. It is interesting that at a time when in Britain the government departments have shown increased concern that the sponsor of research should get his money's worth in relevant goods, there seems also to be a groundswell of demand from all manner of social workers and people 'out there' that research should be relevant also to the needs of their particular sector of the front line. The research worker suddenly discovers that the world is rather reluctant to subsidise what it perceives to be a luxury trade. The worth of fundamental and theoretical research is sometimes misunderstood, but that is largely not what is under attack.

The message carried by this set of papers would therefore seem to be that in an era of questioning, there must be live and intelligent scrutiny both of the inner workings of any research group and at the same time of the nature and import of the many outside relationships which should feed on awareness of what research is to be done, and of how research findings are to be made useful and intelligible to the many interests which together constitute the range of potential consumers. These questions are very easily for ever left lying around, but it is time that the research world got beyond the stage of vague guilt and determined that these issues should no longer be treated as optional extras to the generation of data.

The final appraisal of this section properly rounds off the book itself. In part the challenge which is identified is that of continuously ensuring that in this particularly difficult scientific field the right questions are asked, the best methods for their scientific solution deployed by the team, the most economical methods of analysis utilised, the findings properly related to the literature. But the research sections and the section on the research position

238

are then brought together by that remark of Toynbee's which is quoted in the paper by Timothy Cook – the ultimate challenge is still 'to make benevolence scientific'.

List of contributors

Cole, P., FFARCS, Anaesthetics Laboratory, St. Bartholomew's Hospital, London.

Cook, T., MA, Alcoholics Recovery Project, London.

Edwards, G., MA, DM, MRCP, MRC Psych., Hon. Director, Addiction Research Unit; Reader in Drug Dependence, Institute of Psychiatry; Hon. Consultant Psychiatrist, Bethlem Royal and Maudsley Hospitals.

Falkowski, W., MB, BCh, MRCGP, DPM, MPhil, MRC Psych., Hon. Consultant Psychiatrist, St. George's Hospital, London.

Gath, D., MA, DM, MRCP, MRC Psych., First Assistant, Oxford University Department of Psychiatry; Hon. Consultant Psychiatrist, Warneford Hospital, Oxford and United Oxford Hospitals.

Gattoni, F., MSc., Associate Lecturer, Department of Humanities, University of Surrey.

Gelder, M. G., MA, DM, FRCP, FRC Psych., Professor of Psychiatry, Department of Psychiatry, University of Oxford.

Guthrie, S., MA, *formerly* research social worker, Addiction Research Unit.

Hawker, A., Medical Council on Alcoholism, London; *formerly* research worker, Addiction Research Unit.

Hawks, D. V., BA, Postgrad.Dip.Psychol., PhD, Senior Clinical Psychologist, Department of Clinical Psychology, Whitchurch Hospital, Wales; *formerly* Deputy Director and Senior Lecturer, Addiction Research Unit.

Hensman, C., MA, Soc.Sc.Dip., Regional Principal, DHSS; *formerly* research social worker and research administrator, Addiction Research Unit.

Hore, B. D., BSc, MB, MRCP, MPhil., Consultant-in-Charge, Alcoholism Treatment Unit, Springfield Hospital, Manchester.

Kelly, M. G., MD, MRC Psych., DPM, Medical Director, Drug Advisory and Treatment Centre, Jervis Street Hospital, Dublin.

MacCafferty, M. M. P., BSc, ALA, A.Inst.Inf.Sc., Information Scientist and Chartered Librarian, Addiction Research Unit.

Nicholls, P., MSc, Lecturer, Biometrics Unit, Institute of Psychiatry.

Ogborne, A. C., MSc, PhD, Addiction Research Foundation; *formerly* Lecturer, Addiction Research Unit.

Orford, J., MA, Dip.Psychol., Lecturer, Addiction Research Unit.

Peto, J., MA, MSc, DIC, Research Officer, DHSS Cancer Epidemiological and Clinical Trials Unit, University of Oxford; *formerly* research worker, Addiction Research Unit.

Pollak, B., MRCGP, Honorary Tutor, General Practice, St. Thomas's Medical School, London; Clinical assistant, Maudsley Hospital; Medical Advisor, Alcoholics Recovery Project, London.

Russell, M. A. H., BM, MRCP, MRC Psych., Hon. Consultant Psychiatrist, Maudsley Hospital; Senior Lecturer, Addiction Research Unit.

Spratley, T. A., MB, BS, MRCP, MPhil., MRC Psych., Maudsley Alcoholism Pilot Project, Maudsley Hospital.

Waller, S. (née Postoyan), BA, Dip.Soc.Admin., *formerly* research worker, Addiction Research Unit.

Williamson, V., MA, *formerly* research worker, Addiction Research Unit.

References

Adamson, J. D., and Schmale, A. H., 'Object loss, giving up, and the onset of psychiatric disease', *Psychosomatic Medicine,* vol. 27 (1965), pp. 557–76.

Aitken, R. C. B., 'Measurement of feelings using visual analogue scales', *Proceedings of the Royal Society of Medicine.,* vol. 62 (1969), pp. 989–93.

Armstrong, W., 'The view from the government', Social Science Research Council Newsletter, no. 7 (December 1969).

Ashton, H., Watson, D. W., Marsh, R., and Sadler, J., 'Puffing frequency and nicotine intake in cigarette smokers', *British Medical Journal,* vol. 3 (1970), pp. 679–81.

Astrup, P., 'Some physiological and pathological effects of moderate carbon monoxide exposure', *British Medical Journal,* vol. 4 (1972), pp. 447–52.

Bahn, A. K., Anderson, C. L., and Norman, V. B., 'Outpatient psychiatric clinic services to alcoholics', *Quarterly Journal of Studies on Alcohol,* vol. 24 (1963), pp. 213–26.

Bailey, M. B., Haberman, P., and Alksne, H., 'Outcome of alcoholic marriages: endurance, termination of recovery', *Quarterly Journal of Studies on Alcohol,* vol. 23 (1962), pp. 610–23.

Ball, K., 'Hospital beds and cigarette smoking', *Lancet,* vol. 2 (1970), p. 48.

Beard, R. R., and Grandstaff, N., 'Carbon monoxide exposure and cerebral function', Annals of the New York Academy of Sciences, vol. 174 (1970), pp. 385–95.

Berglund, E., 'Tobacco withdrawal clinics', Norwegian Cancer Society (1969).

Bill, C., 'The growth and effectiveness of Alcoholics Anonymous in a south-western city, 1945–1962', *Quarterly Journal of Studies on Alcohol,* vol. 26 (1965), pp. 279–84.

Blom, A., 'Some experience regarding the use of metronidazole in the treatment of alcoholism', *Svenska Lakartidninger,* vol. 64 (1967), pp. 57–61.

Bonfiglio, G., and Donadio, G., 'Results of the clinical testing of a new drug "Metronidazole" in the treatment of chronic alcoholism', *British Journal of Addiction,* vol. 62 (1967), pp. 249–55.

Boulding, K., 'Dare one take the social sciences seriously?' *American Psychology,* vol. 22 (1967), pp. 879–87.

Bowden, C. H., and Woodhall, W. R., 'The determination and significance of low blood carboxyhaemoglobin levels', *Medical Science and Law,* vol. 4

(1964), pp. 98–107.

British Medical Journal: 'Down and out', vol. 2 (1966), p. 1546.

British Medical Journal: 'Treating the drunken offender', vol. 2 (1968), pp. 505–6.

Brown G. W. and Birley, J. L. T., 'Crises and life changes and the onset of schizophrenia', *Journal of Health and Social Behaviour,* vol. 9 (1968), pp. 203–14.

Bruun, K., 'Outcome of different types of treatment of alcoholics', *Quarterly Journal of Studies on Alcohol,* vol. 24 (1963), pp. 280–8.

Bynner, J. M., 'The young smoker', Government Social Survey, HMSO, London (1969).

Camberwell Council on Alcoholism, 'The Chronic Drunkenness Offender: a therapeutic alternative to repeated imprisonment', London (1965), unpublished.

Cartwright, A., Martin, F. M., and Thomson, J. G., 'Efficacy of an anti-smoking campaign', *Lancet,* vol. 1 (1960), pp. 327–9.

Cassidy, W. L., Flanagan, N. B., Spilliman, M., and Cohen, M. E., 'Clinical observations in manic depressive disease', *Journal of the American Medical Association,* vol. 164 (1957), pp. 1535–46.

Central Statistical Office: *Annual abstract of statistics,* no. 106, HMSO, London (1969).

Central Statistical Office: *Statistical Digest of the War,* HMSO, London (1951).

Central Statistical Office (1971a): 'The internal purchasing power of the pound', *Statistical News* (May 1971), no. 13, pp. 14–7, HMSO, London. (Updated figures in pamphlet on 'Internal Purchasing Power of the Pound' (20 October 1972), circulated by the Central Statistical Office). CSO (1971b): Figures for 1960–70 in *Economic Trends,* no. 216 (October 1971), table 8, p. 53, HMSO, London. (Figures for the other years were supplied by the Central Statistical Office).

Chafetz, M. E., 'A procedure for establishing therapeutic contact with the alcoholic', *Quarterly Journal of Studies on Alcohol,* vol. 22 (1961), pp. 325–28.

Chandler, J., Hensman, C., and Edwards, G., 'Determinants of what happens to alcoholics', *Quarterly Journal of Studies on Alcohol,* vol. 32 (1971), pp. 349–63.

Cherns, A. B., 'Putting Psychology to Work', *Occupational Psychology,* vol. 41 (1967), pp. 77–84.

Cherns, A. B., 'Relation between Research Institutions and Users of Research', *International Social Science Journal,* vol. 22 (1970), pp. 226–42.

Cherns, A. B., 'Social Psychology and Development', *Bulletin of British Psychological Society,* vol. 22 (1969), pp. 93–7.

Cherns, A. B., 'The use of the Social Sciences', *Human Relations,* vol. 21 (1968), pp. 313–25.

Coburn, R. F., Forster, R. E., and Kane, P. B., 'Consideration of the physiological variables that determine the blood carboxyhemoglobin concentration in man', *Journal of Clinical Investigation,* vol. 44 (1965), p. 1899.

Commins, B. T., and Lawther, P. J., 'A sensitive method for the determination of carboxyhaemoglobin in a finger prick sample of blood', *British Journal of Industrial Medicine,* vol. 22 (1965), pp. 139–43.

Cook, T., Gath, D., and Hensman, C., *The Drunkenness Offence,* Pergamon Press, Oxford (1969).

Cook, T., Morgan, H. G., and Pollak, B., 'The Rathcoole Experiment: first year at a hostel for vagrant alcoholics', *British Medical Journal,* vol. 1 (1968), pp. 240–2.

Cooper, J., and Maule, H. G., 'Problems of drinking: an enquiry among members of "Alcoholics Anonymous" ', *British Journal of Addiction,* vol. 58, (1962), pp. 45–53.

Davies, D. L., 'Normal drinking in recovered alcohol addicts', *Quarterly Journal of Studies on Alcohol,* vol. 23 (1962), pp. 94–104.

Davies, D. L., Shepherd, M., and Myers, E., 'The two-years' prognosis of 50 alcohol addicts after treatment in hospital', *Quarterly Journal of Studies on Alcohol,* vol. 17 (1956), pp. 485–501.

Department of Health and Social Security: 'Report of the Standing Scientific Liaison Committee to the Secretary of State for Social Services on the publication of tar and nicotine yields of packeted cigarettes', DHSS, London (1973).

Doll, R., and Hill, A. B., 'Smoking and carcinoma of the lung: preliminary report', *British Medical Journal,* vol. 2 (1950), pp. 739–48.

Dorfman, R., *The Price System,* Prentice–Hall, New Jersey (1964).

Edwards, G., 'Epidemiology applied to alcoholism. A review and an examination of purpose', *Quarterly Journal of Studies on Alcohol,* vol. 34 (1973), pp. 28–56.

Edwards, G., 'Hypnosis in treatment of alcohol addiction. Controlled trial, with analysis of factors affecting outcome', *Quarterly Journal of Studies on Alcohol,* vol. 27 (1966), pp. 221–41.

Edwards, G., 'Unreason in an age of reason: past history and present mental state', Edwin Stevens Lecture (1971), Royal Society of Medicine, London.

Edwards, G., and Guthrie, S., 'A comparison of inpatient and outpatient treatment of alcohol dependence', *Lancet,* vol. 2 (1966), pp. 467–8.

Edwards, G. and Jaffe, J. H., Working paper prepared for the WHO expert committee on drug dependence, Geneva (August 1970), unpublished.

Edwards, G., Gattoni, F., and Hensman, C., 'Correlates of alcohol – dependence scores in a prison population', *Quarterly Journal of Studies on Alcohol,* vol. 33 (1972), pp. 417–29.

Edwards, G., Hawker, A., and Hensman, C., 'Setting up a therapeutic community', *Lancet,* vol. 2 (1966a), pp. 1407–8.

Edwards, G., Hensman, C., and Peto, J., 'A comparison of female and male motivation for drinking', *International Journal of the Addictions,* vol. 8 (1974), pp. 577–87.

Edwards, G., Hawker, A., Williamson, V., and Hensman, C., 'London's Skid Row', *Lancet,* vol. 1 (1966b), pp. 249–52.

Edwards, G., Hensman, C., Chandler, J., and Peto, J., 'Motivation for drinking among men: survey of a London suburb', *Psychological Medicine,* vol. 2 (1972d), pp. 260–71.

Edwards, G., Williamson, V., Hawker, A., Hensman, C., and Postoyan, S., 'Census of a reception centre', *British Journal of Psychiatry,* vol. 114 (1968), pp. 1031–39.

Evans, M., Fine, E., and Phillips, W. Powell, 'Community care for alcoholics and their families', *British Medical Journal,* vol. 1 (1966), pp. 1531–2.

Eysenck, H. J., *Manual of the Maudsley Personality Inventory,* University of London Press (1959).

Eysenck, H. J., *Smoking, Health and Personality,* Weidenfeld and Nicolson, London (1965).

Eysenck, S. B. G., and Eysenck, H. J., 'An improved short questionnaire for the measurement of extroversion and neuroticism', *Life Sciences,* vol. 3 (1964), pp. 1103–9.

Forrest, A. D., Fraser, R. N., and Priest, R. G., 'Environmental factors in Depressive Illness', *British Journal of Psychiatry,* vol. 111 (1965), pp. 243–53.

Frith, C. D., 'The effect of varying the nicotine content of cigarettes on human smoking behaviour', *Psychopharmacologia,* vol. 19 (1971), pp. 188–92.

Gath, D., Hensman, C., Hawker, A., Kelly, M., and Edwards, G., 'The Drunk in Court: Survey of Drunkenness Offenders from Two London Courts', *British Medical Journal,* vol. 4 (1968), pp. 808–11.

General Register Office: *Classification of Occupations, 1960,* HMSO, London.

General Register Office: *Classification of Occupations, 1966,* HMSO, London.

Giffen, P. J., Personal communications from Alcoholism and Drug Addiction

Research Foundation of Ontario, Canada (1966–68).

Glatt, M., 'Drinking habits of English (middle class) alcoholics', *Acta Psychiatrica Scandinavica,* vol. 37 (1961a), pp. 88–113.

Glatt, M., 'Treatment results in an English mental hospital alcoholic unit', *Acta Psychiatrica Scandinavica,* vol. 37 (1961b), pp. 143–68.

Godber, G., 'It can be done' in R. G. Richardson (ed.), *The Second World Conference on Smoking and Health, 1971,* Pitman's Medical Publishers, London (1972), pp. 141–7.

Godber, G. E., 'On the state of the public health. The annual report of the chief medical officer of the Ministry of Health for the year 1968', HMSO, London (1969), p. 226.

Godber, G. E., 'On the state of the public health. The annual report of the chief medical officer of the Ministry of Health for the year 1969', HMSO, London (1970a), p. 8.

Godber, G. E., 'Smoking disease: a self-inflicted injury', *American Journal of Public Health,* vol. 60 (1970b), p. 235.

Goldfarb, T. L., and Jarvik, M. E., 'Accommodation to restricted tobacco smoke intake in cigarette smokers', *International Journal of the Addictions,* vol. 7 (1972), pp. 559–65.

Goldfarb, T. L., Jarvik, M. E., and Glick, S. D., 'Cigarette nicotine content as a determinant of human smoking behavior', *Psychopharmacologia,* vol. 17 (1970), pp. 89–93.

Goldsmith, J. R., 'Contribution of motor vehicle exhaust, industry, and cigarette smoking to community carbon monoxide exposures', Annals of New York Academy of Sciences, vol. 174 (1970), pp. 122–34.

Great Britain, Laws, Statutes: Criminal Justice Act, 1967, HMSO, London (1968).

Halsey, A. H., *Educational Priority: report of a research project sponsored by the DES and the SSRC., vol. 1: EPA problems and policies,* HMSO, London (1972).

Hammond, E. C., 'Smoking in relation to the death rates of one million men and women', *National Cancer Institute Monogram,* vol. 19 (1966), pp. 127–204.

Hare, E. H., and Shaw, G. K., 'Mental health on a new housing estate', Maudsley Monograph 12, Oxford University Press, London (1965).

von Harke, H. P., 'Zum Problem des "Passiv-Rauchens" ', *Münchener Medizinische Wochenschrift,* vol. 112 (1970), pp. 2328–34.

Hawkins, L. H., *Journal of Scientific Technology,* vol. 13 (1967), p. 21.

Hendrickson, A. E., and White, P. O., 'Promax: a quick method for rotation to oblique simple structure', *British Journal of Statistical Psychology,* vol. 17 (1964), pp. 65–70.

246

HM Customs and Excise annual reports, HMSO, London (1967–70).

Higbee, K. L., 'Fifteen years of fear arousal: research on threat appeals 1953–1968', *Psychological Bulletin,* vol. 72 (1969), pp. 426–44.

Hill, A. B., 'The environment and disease: association or causation?', *Proceedings Royal Society of Medicine,* vol. 58 (1965), pp. 295–300.

Holland, W. W., and Elliott, A., 'Cigarette smoking, respiratory symptoms, and anti-smoking propaganda', *Lancet,* vol. 1 (1968), pp. 41–3.

Home Office: 'Offences of Drunkenness, 1967', Cmnd. 3663, HMSO, London (1968).

Hore, B. D., 'Factors in Alcoholic Relapse', *British Journal of Addiction,* vol. 66 (1971), pp. 83–8.

Hudgens, R. W., Morrison, J. R., and Barchha, R. G., 'Life events and onset of primary affective symtoms. A study of 40 hospitalized patients and 40 controls', *Archives of General Psychiatry,* vol. 16 (1967), pp. 134–45.

Jackson, J. K., 'The adjustment of the family to the crisis of alcoholism', *Quarterly Journal of Studies on Alcohol,* vol. 15 (1954), pp. 562–86.

Jeffreys, M., Norman-Taylor, W., and Griffith, G., 'Longer term results of an anti-smoking educational campaign', *Medical Officer,* vol. 117 (1967), p. 93.

Jellinek, E. M., *The Disease Concept of Alcoholism,* Hillhouse Press, New Haven (1960).

Jellinek, E. M., Harris, I., Lundquist, G., Tiebout, H. M., Duchene, H., Mardones, J., and MacLeod, L. D., 'The "craving" for alcohol. A symposium by members of the WHO Expert Committees on Mental Health and on Alcohol', *Quarterly Journal of Studies on Alcohol,* vol. 16 (1955), pp. 34–66.

Jones, R. D., Commins, B. T., and Cernik, A. A., 'Blood lead and carboxyhaemoglobin levels in London taxi drivers', *Lancet,* vol. 2 (1972), pp. 302–3.

Kendell, R. E., 'Normal drinking by former alcohol addicts', *Quarterly Journal of Studies on Alcohol,* vol. 26 (1965), pp. 247–57.

Lancet: 'Tar and nicotine yields of cigarettes', vol. 1 (1973), pp. 874–5.

Lawley, D. N., and Maxwell, A. E., *Factor analysis as a statistical method,* Butterworths, London (1963).

Lawther, P. J., and Commins, B. T., 'Cigarette smoking and exposure to carbon monoxide', *Annals of the New York Academy of Sciences,* vol. 174 (1970) pp. 135–47.

Lazarus, R. S., *Psychological stress and the coping process,* McGraw-Hill, New York (1966).

Lemert, E. M., 'The occurrence and sequence of events in the adjustment of families to alcoholism', *Quarterly Journal of Studies on Alcohol,* vol. 21

(1960), pp. 679–97.

Lester, D., 'Alcohol self-selection and human variation', *Quarterly Journal of Studies on Alcohol,* vol. 27 (1966), pp. 395–438.

Leventhal, H., 'Experimental studies of anti-smoking communications' in E. F. Borgatta and R. R. Evans (eds), *Smoking, Health and Behavior,* Aldine Publishing Co., Chicago (1968), pp. 95–121.

Lily, R. E. C., Cole, P. V., and Hawkins, L. H., 'Spectrophotometric measurement of carboxyhaemoglobin, an evaluation of the method of Commins and Lawther', *British Journal of Industrial Medicine,* vol. 29 (1972), pp. 454–7.

Lowe, C. R., 'The cost to health of addiction to tobacco', paper presented at International Conference on Alcohol and Addictions, Cardiff, (21–25 September 1970).

McDonald, M. E., 'Social work research: a perspective' in N. A. Polansky (ed.), *Social Work Research,* University of Chicago Press (1960), pp. 1–20.

McKennell, A. C., and Thomas, R. K., 'Adults' and adolescents' smoking habits and attitudes', Government Social Survey, HMSO, London (1967).

Marks, I. M., 'Patterns of Meaning in Psychiatric Patients', Maudsley Monograph 13, Oxford University Press, London (1965).

Marshall, T. H., *Sociology at the Cross Roads and other Essays,* Heinemann, London (1963).

Mayer, J. E., and Timms, N., *The Client Speaks: Working class impressions of case work,* Routledge & Kegan Paul (1970).

Media Expenditure Analysis Ltd.: personal communication (1970).

Ministry of Health: First report of the Interdepartmental Committee on Drug Addiction, HM 62 43, HMSO (1962).

Morris, J. N., *Uses of Epidemiology,* Livingstone, Edinburgh, (1957).

Moss, M. C., and Davies, E. B., *A Survey of Alcoholism in an English County,* Geigy Scientific Publications, London (1967).

Myerson, D. J., 'Approach to Skid Row problem in Boston', *New England Journal of Medicine,* vol. 249 (1953), pp. 646–9.

Myerson, D. J., 'The Skid Row problem: further observations on a group of alcoholic patients, with emphasis on interpersonal relations and the therapeutic approach', *New England Journal of Medicine,* vol. 254 (1956), pp. 1168–73.

National Council on Alcoholism: 'The Skid Row Population in the United States and the Incidence of Alcoholism amongst its Habitués', National Council on Alcoholism, New York (1959).

National Council on Alcoholism: 'What you should know about Alcoholism', National Council on Alcoholism, New York (1965).

O'Brien, T. H., *Civil Defence,* HMSO, London (1955).

Oppenheim, A. N. *Questionnaire design and attitude measurement,* Heinemann, London (1966).

Orlans, G., 'Making social research more useful to government', *Social Science Information,* vol. 7 (1968), pp. 151–8.

Park, P., 'Problem drinking and social orientation', an unpublished PhD thesis, Yale University, Connecticut (1958).

Parr, D., 'Offences of drunkenness in the London area: a pilot study', *British Journal of Criminology,* vol. 2 (1962), pp. 272–7.

Perceval, R. 'Information centres on alcoholism', *Medical Officer,* vol. 115 (1966), pp. 59–60.

Pittman, D. J., 'Existing and proposed treatment facilities in the USA, paper presented at International Symposium on "The Drunkenness Offence" ', Institute of Psychiatry, London (1968).

Pittman, D. J., and Gordon, C. W., *The Revolving Door: A Study of the Chronic Police Court Inebriate,* Free Press, Glencoe, Illinois (1958).

Rahe, R. H., 'Life-change measurement as a predictor of illness', *Proceedings of the Royal Society of Medicine,* vol. 61 (1968), pp. 1124–6.

Rathod, N. H., Gregory, E., Blows, D., and Thomas, G. H., 'A two year follow-up study of alcoholic patients', *British Journal of Psychiatry,* vol. 112 (1966), pp. 683–92.

Robinson, D., 'The Alcohologist's addiction, some implications of having lost control over the disease concept of alcoholism', condensed from *Quarterly Journal of Studies on Alcohol,* vol. 33 (1972a), pp. 1028–42.

Robinson, D., Day, I., Edwards, G., Hawks, D., Hershon, H., MacCafferty, M., Oppenheimer, E., Orford, J., Otto, S., and Taylor, C., 'Where Errol went wrong on liquor licensing. A critique of the Report of the Departmental Committee on Liquor Licensing, Cmnd. 5154, HMSO (1972)', Camberwell Council on Alcoholism (1973).

Royal College of Physicians' Report: *Smoking and Health,* Pitman Medical Publishing Co. Ltd., London (1962).

Royal College of Physicians: *Smoking and Health Now,* Pitman Medical Publishing Co. Ltd., London (1971).

Russell, C. S., Taylor, R., and Maddison, R. N., 'Some effects of smoking in pregnancy', *Journal of Obstetrics and Gynaecology of the British Commonwealth,* vol. 73 (1966), pp. 742–6.

Russell, M. A. H., comment in *The Second World Conference on Smoking and Health,* edited by R. G. Richardson, Pitman Medical Publishing Co. Ltd., London (1972), p. 52.

Russell, M. A. H., 'Cigarette Dependence: II– Doctor's role in Management', *British Medical Journal,* vol. 2 (1971c), pp. 393–5.

Russell, M. A. H. 'Cigarette smoking: natural history of a dependence disorder', *British Journal Medical Psychology,* vol. 44 (1971a), pp. 1–16.

Russell, M. A. H., 'Effect of Electric Aversion on Cigarette Smoking', synopsis of a paper of the same title which originally appeared in *British Medical Journal,* vol. 1 (1970), pp. 82–6.

Russell, M. A. H., 'Tobacco and the Nation's Health' in J. Zacune and C. Hensman (eds) *Drugs, Alcohol and Tobacco in Britain: The problems and the response* (1971b), pp. 211–9.

Russell, M. A. H., Cole, P. V., and Brown, E., 'Absorption by non-smokers of carbon monoxide from room air polluted by tobacco smoke', *Lancet,* vol. 1 (1973b), pp. 576–9.

Russell, M. A. H., Wilson, C., Cole, P. V., Idle, M., and Feyerabend, C., 'Comparison of increases in carboxyhaemoglobin after smoking "extra-mild" and "non-mild" cigarettes', *Lancet,* vol. 2 (1973a), pp. 687–690.

Samuelson, P. A., *Economics: An Introductory Analysis,* 7th edition, McGraw-Hill, New York (1967).

Schwartz, J. L., 'A critical review and evaluation of smoking control methods', Public Health Reports 84, 483 (1969).

Semer, J. M., Friedland, P., Vaisberg, M., and Greenberg, A., 'The Use of metronidazole in the treatment of alcoholism: a pilot study', *American Journal of Psychiatry,* vol. 123 (1966), pp. 722–4.

Shields, J., 'Monozygotic twins brought up apart and brought up together: an investigation into the genetic and environmental causes of variations in personality', Oxford University Press (1962).

Shyne, A. W., use of available material, ch. 6 in N. A. Polansky (ed.), *Social Work Research,* University of Chicago Press (1960).

Social Science Research Council: Annual Report 1969–70, HMSO, London (1970).

Social Science Research Council: 'Research and Government', *Newsletter* no. 7 (December 1969).

Srch, M. 'Über die Bedeutung des Kohlenoxyds beim Zigarettenrauchen im Personenkraftwageninneren', *Deutsche Zeitschrift für Gerichtliche Medizin,* vol. 60 (1967), pp. 80–9.

Stone, R., *The Measurement of Consumers' Expenditure and Behaviour in the United Kingdom 1920–1938,* vol. 1, University Press, Cambridge (1954).

Straus, R., 'Alcohol and the homeless man', *Quarterly Journal of Studies on Alcohol,* vol. 7 (1946), pp. 360–404.

Straus, R., and Bacon, S. D., *Drinking in College,* Yale University Press, New Haven, Connecticut (1953).

250

Straus, R., and McCarthy, R. G., 'Nonaddictive pathological drinking patterns of homeless men', *Quarterly Journal of Studies on Alcohol*, vol. 12 (1951), pp. 601–11.

Tobacco Trade Year Book and Diary 1972, edited by V. Raven, International Trade Publications Ltd., London.

Todd, G. F., *Statistics of Smoking in the United Kingdom 1972*, Tobacco Research Council.

Turner, M. L., occasional reports: *The halfway house, The second house, Safe lodging, The lessons of Norman House, Second House*, Norman House, London (1964–68).

US Department of Health, Education and Welfare: Report of the Surgeon General, *The Health Consequences of Smoking* (1972).

US National Air Pollution Control Administration: 'Air Quality Criteria for Carbon Monoxide', US Government Printing Office, Washington, DC (1970).

Vallance, M., 'Alcoholism. A two-year follow-up study of patients admitted to the psychiatric department of a general hospital', *British Journal of Psychiatry*, vol. 111 (1965), pp. 348–56.

Victor, M., and Adams, R. D., 'The effect of alcohol on the nervous system', *Association for Research into Nervous and Mental Diseases*, vol. 32 (1953), pp. 526–73.

Waingrow, S., and Horn, D., 'Relationship of number of cigarettes smoked to "tar" rating', National Cancer Institute Monograms, vol. 28 (1968), pp. 29–33.

Wallerstein, R. S., *Hospital Treatment of Alcoholism*, Menninger Clinic Monograph, no. 11, Imago, London (1957).

Walton, H. J., Ritson, E. B. and Kennedy, R. I., 'Response of alcoholics to clinic treatment', *British Medical Journal*, vol. 2 (1966), pp. 1171–4.

Watson, P., 'Social Sciences: Research Priorities', *New Society*, (13 August 1970).

Wikler, A., 'Interaction of physical dependence and classical and operant conditions in the genesis of relapse' in *The Addictive States*, vol. 46 of Association for Research in Nervous and Mental Disease, Williams and Wilkins, Baltimore, (1968), pp. 280–7.

Wikler, A., 'On the nature of addiction and habituation', *British Journal of Addiction*, vol. 57 (1961), pp. 73–9.

Wing, J., *Community Psychiatric Services*, Oxford University Press (1973).

Wootton, B., *In a World I Never Made*, Allen and Unwin, London (1967).

Wootton, B., *Social Science and Social Pathology*, Allen and Unwin, London (1959).

Wynder, E. L., contribution in R. G. Richardson (ed.), *The Second World*

Conference on Smoking and Health, Pitman Medical Publishing Co. Ltd., London (1972), pp. 197–8.

Wynder, E. L. and Hoffman, D., 'Tobacco and tobacco smoke. Studies in experimental carcinogenesis', Academic Press, New York (1967), p. 443.

Zax, M., Gardner, E. A. and Hart, W. T., 'Public intoxication in Rochester. A survey of individuals charged during 1961', *Quarterly Journal of Studies on Alcohol,* vol. 25 (1964), pp. 669–78.

Bibliography of the Addiction Research Unit

Blumberg, H. H., 'British users of opiate-type drugs: a follow-up study', *British Journal of Addiction* (in press).

Blumberg, H. H., 'Drug taking among children and adolescents' in M. Rutter and L. Hersov (eds) *Recent Developments in Child Psychiatry*, Oxford in press), ch. 23.

Blumberg, H. H., 'Professional education and training on the problems of alcohol and drugs' in J. Zacune and C. Hensman (eds) *Drugs, Alcohol and Tobacco in Britain*, London (1971), ch. 18.

Blumberg, H. H., 'Surveys of drug use among young people', *International Journal of the Addictions* (in press).

Blumberg, H. H., Cohen, S. D., Dronfield, B. E., Mordecai, E. A., Roberts, J. C., and Hawks, D. V., 'British opiate users: I People approaching London drug treatment centres' *International Journal of the Addictions*, vol. 9 (1974), pp. 1–23.

Blumberg, H. H., Cohen, S. D., Dronfield, B. E., Mordecai, E. A., Roberts, J. C., and Hawks, D. V., 'British opiate users: II Difference between those given an opiate script and those not given one', *International Journal of the Addictions*, vol. 9 (1974), pp. 205–20.

Blumberg, H. H., Cohen, S. D., Dronfield, B. E., Mordecai, E. A., Roberts, J. C., and Hawks, D. V., 'Opiate use in London', *Journal of the American Medical Association* (in press).

Chandler, J., Hensman, C., and Edwards, G., 'Determinants of what happens to alcoholics', *Quarterly Journal of Studies on Alcohol*, vol. 32 (1971), pp. 349–63.

Crow, I., 'Two groups of cannabis users in South London', *Drugs & Society*, vol. 2 (June 1973), pp. 10–14.

Edwards, G., 'Addiction as a public health problem', *Medical Officer*, vol. 113 (1965), pp. 177–80.

Edwards, G., 'Alcoholic swamps', *New Society*, vol. 2 (September 1971), pp. 459–61.

Edwards, G., 'Alcoholism as a public health problem in the USA', *Lancet*, vol. 1 (1962), pp. 960–2.

Edwards, G., 'Alcoholism studies and the Addiction Research Unit' in *Portfolio for Health. 2 The developing programme of the DHSS in health services research*. DHSS, London (1973).

Edwards, G., 'Alternative strategies for minimizing alcohol problems: coming out of the doldrums', *Journal of Alcoholism* (in press).

Edwards, G., 'The British approach to the treatment of heroin addiction', *Lancet*, vol. 1 (1969), pp. 768–72.

Edwards, G., 'Cannabis and the criteria for legislation of a currently prohibited recreational drug: groundwork for a debate', *Acta Psychiatrica Scandinavica*, supplementum 251 (1974), pp. 1–62.

Edwards, G., 'Cannabis and the psychiatric position' in J. D. P. Graham (ed.) *Cannabis sativa*, London (in press).

Edwards, G., 'The circulating alcoholic', *Medicine, Science and the Law* (October 1964), pp. 254–8.

Edwards, G., 'Classification of pathological drinking', paper presented at Third Symposium on Advanced Medicine held at the Royal College of Physicians, London, February 1967; proceedings published by Pitman, London (1967), pp. 303–16.

Edwards, G., 'A community as case study: alcoholism treatment in antiquity and Utopia', paper, 2nd Annual Alcoholism Conference, National Institute on Alcohol Abuse and Alcoholism, Washington DC (June 1972), pp. 1–2.

Edwards, G., 'Double-blind trial of lobeline in an anti-smoking clinic', *Medical Officer*, vol. 112 (1964), pp. 158–60.

Edwards, G., 'A doubtful prognosis', *International Journal of Psychiatry*, vol. 9, (1970–71), pp. 354–8.

Edwards, G., 'Drug dependence – putting history on the agenda', paper, Round Table Conference on Non-medical Use of Dependence-producing Drugs, Geneva (1971).

Edwards, G., 'Drug problems UK/USA', *Proceedings of the Royal Society of Medicine* (1973), pp. 2–6.

Edwards, G., 'Drugs, drug dependence and the concept of plasticity', *Quarterly Journal of Studies on Alcohol*, vol. 35 (1974), pp. 176–95.

Edwards, G., 'The early diagnosis of alcoholism', *Medical World* (November 1961), pp. 372–6.

Edwards, G., 'Encounter with the alcoholic', *Medical World* (December 1960), pp. 512–18.

Edwards, G., 'Epidemiology applied to alcoholism. A review and an examination of purposes', *Quarterly Journal of Studies on Alcohol*, vol. 34 (1973), pp. 28–56.

Edwards, G., 'Hypnosis and lobeline in an anti-smoking clinic', *Medical Officer*, vol. 111 (1964), pp. 239–43.

Edwards, G., 'Hypnosis in the treatment of alcohol addiction', *Quarterly Journal of Studies on Alcohol*, vol. 27 (1966), pp. 221–41.

Edwards, G., 'The meaning and treatment of alcohol dependence', *Hospital Medicine*, vol. 2 (1967), pp. 272–81.

Edwards, G., 'Patients with drinking problems', *British Medical Journal*, vol. 4 (1968), pp. 435–7.

Edwards, G., 'Personality and addiction', *Howard League Journal*, vol. 12 (1966), pp. 136–9.

Edwards, G., 'Personal view', *British Medical Journal*, vol. 4 (1971), p. 619.

Edwards, G., 'The place of treatment professions in society's response to chemical abuse', *British Medical Journal*, vol. 2 (1970), pp. 195–9.

Edwards, G., 'Planning for the 70's. Social background to the use and abuse of alcohol and drugs; professional aspects', in *Proceedings 29th International Congress on Alcoholism and Drug Dependence*, Sydney (1971).

Edwards, G., 'The problem of cannabis dependence', *Practitioner*, vol. 200 (1968), pp. 226–33.

Edwards, G., 'Public health implications for liquor control', *Lancet*, vol. 2 (1971), pp. 424–5.

Edwards, G., 'The relevance of the American experience of narcotic addiction to the British scene', *British Medical Journal*, vol. 3 (1967), pp. 425–9.

Edwards, G., 'Research report: The Addiction Research Unit of the Institute of Psychiatry, London', *Psychological Medicine*, vol. 2 (1972), pp. 192–7.

Edwards, G., 'The status of alcoholism as a disease', in R. Phillipson (ed.) *Modern Trends in Drug Dependence and Alcoholism*, Butterworth, London (1970).

Edwards, G., 'The streets of Calcutta', *New Society* (7 May 1970), pp. 771–4.

Edwards, G., 'Unreason in the age of reason': I   Past history and present mental state, II   Internal audit; Edwin Stevens Lectures delivered to the Royal Society of Medicine 1971, Royal Society of Medicine, London (1971).

Edwards, G., and Guthrie, S., 'A comparison of in-patient and out-patient treatment of alcohol dependence', *Lancet*, vol. 1 (1966), pp. 467–8.

Edwards, G., and Guthrie, S., 'A controlled trial of in-patient and out-patient treatment of alcohol dependence', *Lancet*, vol. 1 (1967), pp. 555–9.

Edwards, G., Chandler, J., and Hensman, C., 'Drinking in a London suburb: I   Correlates of normal drinking', *Quarterly Journal of Studies on Alcohol*, suppl. 6 (1972), pp. 69–93.

Edwards, G., Gattoni, F., and Hensman, C., 'Correlates of alcohol-dependence scores in a prison population', *Quarterly Journal of Studies on Alcohol*, vol. 33 (1972), pp. 417–29.

Edwards, G., Hawker, A., and Hensman, C., 'Setting up a therapeutic community', *Lancet*, vol. 2 (1966), pp. 1407–8.

Edwards, G., Hensman, C., and Peto, J., 'A comparison of female and male motivation for drinking', *International Journal of the Addictions*, vol. 8, 4

(1974), pp. 577–87.

Edwards, G., Hensman, C., and Peto, J., 'Drinking in a London suburb: III Comparisons of drinking troubles, among men and women', *Quarterly Journal of Studies on Alcohol,* Supplement 6 (1972), pp. 120–8.

Edwards, G., Hensman, C., and Peto, J., 'Drinking in a London suburb: re-interview of a sub-sample and assessment of consistency in answering', *Quarterly Journal of Studies on Alcohol,* vol. 34 (1973), pp. 1244–54.

Edwards, G., Hensman, C., and Peto, J., 'Drinking problems amongst recidivist prisoners', *Psychological Medicine,* vol. 1 (1971), pp. 388–99.

Edwards, G., Kyle, E., and Nicholls, P., 'A study of alcoholics admitted to four hospitals: I Social class and the interaction of the alcoholic with the treatment system', *Quarterly Journal of Studies on Alcoholism,* vol. 35 (1974), pp. 499–522.

Edwards, G., Chandler, J., Hensman, C., and Peto, J., 'Drinking in a London suburb. II Correlates of trouble with drinking among men', *Quarterly Journal of Studies on Alcohol,* Supplement 6 (1972), pp. 94–119.

Edwards, G., Hawker, A., Williamson, V., and Hensman, C., 'London's Skid Row', *Lancet,* vol. 1 (1966), pp. 249–52.

Edwards, G., Hensman, C., Chandler, J., and Peto, J., 'Motivation for drinking among men: survey of a London suburb', *Psychological Medicine,* vol. 2 (1972), pp. 260–71.

Edwards, G., Hensman, C., Hawker, A., and Williamson, V., 'Alcoholics Anonymous: the anatomy of a self-help group', *Social Psychiatry,* vol. 1 (1967), pp. 195–204.

Edwards, G., Hensman, C., Hawker, A., and Williamson, V., 'Who goes to Alcoholics Anonymous?' *Lancet,* vol. 2 (1966), pp. 382–4.

Edwards, G., Kellog-Fisher, M., Hawker, A., and Hensman, C., 'Clients of Alcoholism Information Centres', *British Medical Journal,* vol. 4 (1967), pp. 346–9.

Edwards, G., Hawker, A., Hensman, C., Peto, J., and Williamson, V., 'Alcoholics known or unknown to agencies: epidemiologial studies in a London suburb', *British Journal of Psychiatry,* vol. 123 (1973), pp. 169–83.

Edwards, G., Rathod, N. H., Thomson, I. G., Kyle, E., and Nicholls, P., 'Case note abstraction: a methodological substudy as a cautionary tale', *International Journal of the Addictions,* vol. 11, no. 3 (1976, in press).

Edwards, G., Williamson, V., Hawker, A., Hensman, C., and Postoyan, S., 'Census of a Reception Centre', *British Journal of Psychiatry,* vol. 114 (1968), pp. 1031–9.

Egert, S., 'Casework intervention with families of alcoholics', paper, International Congress on Alcoholism and Drug Dependence, Amsterdam

(1972).

Feyerabend, C., Levitt, T., and Russell, M. A. H., 'A rapid gas-liquid chromatographic estimation of nicotine in biological fluids', *Journal of Pharmacy and Pharmacology* (in press).

Gath, D., Hensman, C., Hawker, A., Kelly, M., and Edwards, G., 'The drunk in court: a survey of drunkenness offenders from two London courts', *British Medical Journal*, vol. 4 (1968), pp. 808–11.

Gelder, M. G., and Edwards, G., 'Metronidazole in the treatment of alcohol addiction: a controlled trial', *British Journal of Psychiatry*, vol. 114 (1968), pp. 437–75.

Hawker, A., Edwards, G., and Hensman, C., 'Problem drinkers on the payroll', *Medical Officer*, vol. 118 (1967), pp. 313–5.

Hawks, D., 'The dimensions of drug dependence in the United Kingdom', *International Journal of the Addictions*, vol. 6 (1971), pp. 135–60.

Hawks, D., 'Drug dependence – a case in point' in E. Vallance (ed.), *The Limits of State Intervention in the Prevention of Self-destructive Behaviour*, Allen & Unwin, London (in press).

Hawks, D., 'The epidemiology of drug dependence in the United Kingdom', *Bulletin on Narcotics*, vol. 22, no. 3 (1970), pp. 15–24.

Hawks, D., 'The epidemiology of narcotic addiction in the United Kingdom' in E. Josephson and E. E. Carroll (eds), *Drug Use: Epidemiological and Sociological Approaches*, Hemisphere P. C., Washington (1974), pp. 45–63.

Hawks, D., 'The evaluation of measures to deal with drug dependence in the United Kingdom', *Proceedings of the Royal Society of Medicine*, vol. 66 (1973), pp. 113–19.

Hawks, D. V., 'Is treatment economical?' *C.C.A. Journal of Alcoholism*, vol. 2, no. 4 (1971), pp. 34–9.

Hawks, D. V., 'Social research as a determinant of social policy', Proceedings of the Second International Institute on the Prevention and Treatment of Drug Dependence, ICAA, Baden (1971).

Hawks, D., Ogborne, A., and Mitcheson, M., 'The strategy of epidemiological research in drug dependence', *British Journal of Addiction*, vol. 65 (1970), pp. 363–8.

Hawks, D., Mitcheson, M., Ogborne, A., and Edwards, G., 'Abuse of Methylamphetamine', *British Medical Journal*, vol. 2 (1969), pp. 715–21.

Hensman, C., 'Alcoholism – psychosocial aspects', paper presented at Third Symposium on Advanced Medicine; Proceedings published by Pitman, London (1967), pp. 317–27.

Hensman, C., 'Problems of drunkenness amongst male recidivists', Proceedings of International Symposium on the Drunkenness Offence,

Published by Pergamon, Oxford (1969), pp. 35–50.

Hensman, C., Chandler, J., Edwards, G., Hawker, A., and Williamson, V., 'Identifying abnormal drinkers: prevalence estimates by general practitioners and clergymen', *Medical Officer,* vol. 120 (1968), pp. 215–20.

Hershon, H. I., 'Alcoholism and the concept of disease', *British Journal of Addiction,* vol. 69 (1974), pp. 123–31.

Hershon, H. I., 'Alcoholism, physical dependence and disease', comment on 'The alcohologist's addiction', *Quarterly Journal of Studies on Alcohol,* vol. 34 (1973), pp. 506–8.

Hershon, H. I., 'Alcohol withdrawal symptoms: phenomenology and implications', *British Journal of Addiction,* vol. 68 (1973), pp. 295–302.

Hershon, H. I., Cook, T., and Foldes, P., 'What shall we do with the drunkenness offender?', *British Journal of Psychiatry,* vol. 124 (1974), pp. 327–35.

Hitchins, L., Mitcheson, M., Zacune, J., and Hawks, D., 'A two-year follow-up of a cohort of opiate users for a provincial town', *British Journal of Addiction,* vol. 66 (1971), pp. 129–40.

Kosviner, A., 'Prevalence, characteristics and correlates of cannabis use in the UK student population', paper, 3rd International Cannabis Conference, London (1974).

Kosviner, A., 'Psychosocial aspects of cannabis use' in J. D. P. Graham (ed.), *Cannabis sativa,* London (in press).

Kosviner, A., 'Unwanted neighbours: a report of public reaction to setting up a residential rehabilitation programme for ex-addicts', *International Journal of the Addictions,* vol. 8 (1973), pp. 801–8.

Kosviner, A., and Hawks, D., 'Cannabis use amongst British university students: II   Patterns of use and attitudes to use amongst users', *British Journal of Addiction* (in press).

Kosviner, A., Hawks, D. V., and Webb, M. G. T., 'Cannabis use among British university students: I   Prevalence rates and differences between students who have tried cannabis and those who have never tried it', *British Journal of Addiction,* vol. 69 (1974), pp. 35–60.

Kosviner, A., Mitcheson, M., Myers, K., Ogborne, A., Stimson, G., Zacune, J., and Edwards, G., 'Heroin use in a provincial town', *Lancet,* vol. 1 (1968), pp. 1189–92.

Kyle, E., 'Patient role and staff role in a therapeutic community', *Journal of Alcoholism,* vol. 4 (1969), pp. 179–82.

Litman, G. K., 'Behavioral modification techniques in the treatment of alcoholism: a review and critique' in *Research advances in alcohol and drug problems,* vol. 3, Toronto (in press).

Litman, G. K., 'Psychological aspects of alcoholism theory and treatment',

Journal of Alcoholism, vol. 9 (1974), pp. 48–9.

Litman, G. K., 'Stress, affect and craving in alcoholics. The single case as a research strategy', *Quarterly Journal of Studies on Alcohol,* vol. 35 (1974), pp. 131–46.

Melotte, C. J., 'A drugs advisory centre', *Social Work Today,* vol. 5 (1974), p. 281.

Melotte, C., 'A rehabilitation hospital, for drug users: one year's admission', *British Journal of Criminology* (in press).

Melotte, C., and Ogborne, A. C., 'Strategies for the successful follow-up of treated drug abusers', *Journal of Drug Issues,* vol. 5 (1975, in press).

Mitcheson, M., Davidson, J., Hawks, D., Hitchins, L., and Malone, S., 'Sedative abuse by heroin addicts', *Lancet,* vol. 1 (1970), pp. 606–7.

Nicholls, P., Edwards, G., and Kyle, E., 'A study of alcoholics admitted to four hospitals: II   General and cause-specific mortality during follow-up', *Quarterly Journal of Studies on Alcohol,* vol. 35 (1974), pp. 841–55.

Ogborne, A. C., 'Addicts, their associations and behaviour', *Social Science and Medicine,* vol. 8 (1974), pp. 557–65.

Ogborne, A. C., 'Coffee pot pourri', *Drugs and Society,* vol. 2, no. 9 (1973), pp. 6–9.

Ogborne, A. C., 'Two types of heroin reaction', *British Journal of Addiction,* vol. 69 (1974), pp. 171–5.

Ogborne, A. C., and Stimson, G. V., 'A three-year follow-up of a representative sample of heroin addicts', *International Journal of the Addictions,* vol. 10, no. 6 (1975).

Orford, J., 'Alcoholism and marriage: the argument against specialism', *Journal of Studies in Alcoholism* (in press).

Orford, J., 'Aspects of the relationship between alcohol and drug abuse', Proceedings, 29th International Congress on Alcoholism and Drug Dependence, Sydney, Australia; Butterworth Press (1971).

Orford, J., 'A comparison of alcoholics whose drinking is totally uncontrolled and alcoholics whose drinking is mainly controlled', *Behaviour, Research and Therapy,* vol. 11 (1973), pp. 565–76.

Orford, J., 'Controlled drinking in the existing behaviour repertoires of alcohol dependent men', *Journal of Alcoholism,* vol. 9 (1974), pp. 56–8.

Orford, J. F., 'Personality factors in alcoholism: a psychological approach', *Update,* vol. 4, (1972), pp. 1371–8.

Orford, J. F., 'A prospective study of the relationship between marital factors and the outcome of treatment for alcoholism', unpublished PhD thesis, University of London (1975).

Orford, J., 'Prospects for research', Proceedings of International Symposium on the Drunkenness Offence, published by Pergamon, Oxford (1969), pp.

165–73.

Orford, J., 'Psychological approaches to alcoholism', *Update*, vol. 3 (1971), pp. 1005–13.

Orford, J., 'Simplistic thinking about other people as a predictor of early drop-out at an alcoholism halfway house', *British Journal of Medical Psychology*, vol. 47 (1947), pp. 53–63.

Orford, J., and Hawker, A., 'An investigation of an alcoholism rehabilitation halfway house: II The complex question of client motivation', *British Journal of Addiction*, vol. 69 (1974), pp. 315–23.

Orford, J., and Hawker, A., 'A note on the ordering of onset of symptoms in alcohol dependence', *Psychological Medicine*, vol. 4 (1974), pp. 281–8.

Orford, J., Hawker, A., and Nicholls, P., 'An investigation of an alcoholism rehabilitation halfway house: I Type of client and modes of discharge', *British Journal of Addiction*, vol. 69 (1974), pp. 213–24.

Orford, J., Hawker, A., and Nicholls, P., 'An investigation of an alcoholism rehabilitation halfway house: III Reciprocal staff-resident evaluation', *British Journal of Addiction*, vol. 70 (1975, in press).

Orford, J., Hawker, A., and Nicholls, P., 'An investigation of an alcoholism rehabilitation halfway house: IV Attractions of the halfway house for residents', *British Journal of Addiction*, vol. 70 (1975, in press).

Orford, J., Walker, S., and Peto, J., 'Drinking behaviour and attitudes and their correlates among university students in England: I Principal components in the drinking domain; II Personality and social influence; III Sex differences, *Quarterly Journal of Studies on Alcohol*, vol. 35 (1974), pp. 1316–74.

Orford, J., Guthrie, S., Nicholls, P., Oppenheimer, E., Egert, S., and Hensman, C., 'Self-reported coping behaviour of wives of excessive drinkers, and its association with drinking outcome', *Journal of Studies of Alcohol* (in press).

Otto, S., 'Women alcoholics. A special case for treatment', *C.C.A. Journal of Alcoholism*, vol. 3, no. 3 (1974), pp. 25–8.

Raw, M., 'Persuading people to stop smoking', *Behaviour, Research and Therapy*, vol. 13, (1975, in press).

Roberts, C., 'How treatment centres help narcotic addicts', *General Practitioner* (1973), pp. 18–19.

Roberts, J. C., 'West End types', *New Society,* (4 February 1971), pp. 195–6.

Roberts, C., 'What do narcotic addicts think of the drug dependence clinics?', *Drugs and Society,* vol. 2, (February 1973), pp. 16–19.

Robinson, D., 'Alcoholism as a social fact: notes on the sociologist's viewpoint in relation to the proposed study of referral behaviour', *British Journal of Addiction*, vol. 68 (1973), pp. 91–7.

Robinson, D., 'The alcohologist's addiction: some implications of having lost control over the disease concept of alcoholism', *Quarterly Journal of Studies on Alcohol,* vol. 33, (1972), pp. 1028–42.

Robinson, D., 'Becoming an alcoholic: handling referrals to an outpatient department', *Japanese Journal of Studies on Alcohol,* vol. 9, no. 2 (1974), pp. 109–22.

Robinson, D., 'Becoming an alcoholic: notes on a study of procedural definitions', *Journal of Alcoholism,* vol. 8 (1973), pp. 5–12.

Robinson, D., 'Becoming ill', *Journal of Psychosomatic Research,* vol. 18, no. 3 (1974), pp. 277–81.

Robinson, D., 'The Erroll Report: key proposals and public reaction', *British Journal of Addiction,* vol. 69 (1974), pp. 99–104.

Robinson, D., 'Illness and deviance' in A. Wertheimer and M. C. Smith (eds), *Pharmacy Practice: Social and Behavioral Aspects,* University Park Press, Baltimore 1974.

Robinson, D., 'Illness behaviour and children's hospitalization: a schema of parents' attitudes toward authority', *Social Science and Medicine,* vol. 6 (1972b), pp. 447–68.

Robinson, D., *Patients, Practitioners and Medical Care: Aspects of Medical Sociology* Heinemann, London (1973).

Robinson, D., 'Please see and advise: making and handling referrals to an alcoholism outpatient clinic', in M. E. J. Wadsworth and D. Robinson (eds), *Studies in Everyday Medical Life,* London (1976, in press).

Robinson, D., *The Process of Becoming Ill* Routledge and Kegan Paul, London (1971).

Robinson, D., 'Sociological theories of dependence: an illogical notion' in D. Hawks, (ed.) *The Epidemiology of Drug Dependence,* WHO (1973).

Robinson, D., 'To what end? Notes on the treatment of alcoholics', *Japanese Journal of Studies on Alcohol',* vol. 10, no. 1, (1974), pp. 123–39.

Robinson, D., 'Where the Erroll Committee went wrong', *Drugs and Society,* vol. 2 (March 1937), pp. 17–20.

Robinson, D., Day, I., Edwards, G., Hawks, D., Hershon, H., MacCafferty, M., Oppenheimer, E., Orford, J., Otto, S., and Taylor, C., 'Where Erroll went wrong on liquor licensing. A critique of The Report of the Departmental Committee on Liquor Licensing', Cmnd. 5154, HMSO (1972), Camberwell Council on Alcoholism (1973).

Russell, M. A. H., 'Blood carboxyhaemoglobin changes during tobacco smoking', *Postgraduate Medical Journal,* vol. 49 (1973), pp. 684–7.

Russell, M. A. H., 'Changes in cigarette price and consumption by men in Britain, 1946–71: a preliminary analysis', *British Journal of Preventive and Social Medicine,* vol. 27 (1973), pp. 1–7.

Russell, M. A. H., 'Cigarette Dependence: I Nature and classification', *British Medical Journal,* vol. 2 (1971), pp. 330–1.

Russell, M. A. H., 'Cigarette Dependence: II Doctor's role in management', *British Medical Journal,* vol. 2 (1971), pp. 393–5.

Russell, M. A. H., 'Cigarette smoking: natural history of a dependence disorder', *British Journal of Medical Psychology,* vol. 44 (1971), pp. 1–16.

Russell, M. A. H., 'Effect of electric aversion on cigarette smoking', *British Medical Journal,* vol. 1 (1970), pp. 82–6.

Russell, M. A. H, 'A psychiatric perspective' in E. Vallance (ed.) *The Limits of State Intervention in the Prevention of Self-destructive Behaviour,* Allen & Unwin, London (1973).

Russell, M. A. H., 'Realistic goals for smoking and health: a case for safe smoking', *Lancet* (1974), pp. 254–7.

Russell, M. A. H., 'The smoking habit and its classification', *The Practitioner,* vol. 212 (1974), pp. 791–800.

Russell, M. A. H., 'Smoking in Britain: strategy for future emancipation', *British Journal of Addiction,* vol. 66 (1971), pp. 157–66.

Russell, M. A. H., 'The smoking problem', *Nursing Times,* vol. 68 (1972), pp. 601–2 and 653–4.

Russell, M. A. H., 'Tobacco and the nation's health' in J. Zacune and C. Hensman (eds.), *Drugs, Alcohol and Tobacco in Britain: the Problems and the Response,* Heinemann, London (1971).

Russell, M. A. H., and Feyerabend, C., 'Blood and urinary nicotine in non-smokers', *Lancet,* vol. 1 (1975), pp. 179–81.

Russell, M. A. H., Armstrong, E., and Patel, U. A., 'Temporal contiguity in electric aversion therapy for cigarette smoking', *Behavior, Research and Therapy* (in press).

Russell, M. A. H., Cole, P. V., and Brown, E., 'Absorption by non-smokers of carbon monoxide from room air polluted by tobacco smoke', *Lancet,* vol. 1 (1973), pp. 576–9.

Russell, M. A. H., Cole, P. V., and Brown, E., 'Passive smoking: absorption by non-smokers of carbon monoxide from room-air polluted by tobacco smoke', *Postgraduate Medical Journal,* vol. 49 (1973), pp. 688–92.

Russell, M. A. H., Peto, J., and Patel, U. A., 'The classification of smoking by factorial structure of motives', *Journal of the Royal Statistical Society,* Series A (General) vol. 137, no. 3 (1974), pp. 313–46.

Russell, M. A. H., Wilson, G., Cole, P. V., Idle, M., and Feyerabend, C., 'Comparison of increases in carboxyhaemoglobin after smoking "extra-mild" and "non-mild" cigarettes', *Lancet,* vol. 2 (1973), pp. 687–90.

Russell, M. A. H., Wilson, C., Patel, U. A., Cole, P. V., and Feyerabend, C., 'Comparison of the effect on tobacco consumption and carbon monoxide absorption of switching to high and low nicotine cigarettes', *British Medical Journal,* vol. 4 (1973), pp. 512–16.

Russell, M. A. H., Wilson, C., Patel, U. A., Feyerabend, C., and Cole, P. V., 'Plasma nicotine levels after smoking cigarettes with high, medium and low nicotine yields', *British Medical Journal* (in press).

Smart, R. G., and Ogborne, A., 'Losses to the addiction notification system', *British Journal of Addiction,* vol. 69 (1974), pp. 225–30.

Stimson, G. V., 'Drug-taking in the younger generation', *Ditchley Paper* no. 4 (1969), p. 32.

Stimson, G. V., 'Heroin behaviour – diversity among addicts attending London clinics', Irish University Press, London and Dublin (1973).

Stimson, G. V., 'Patterns of behaviour of heroin addicts', *International Journal of the Addictions,* vol. 7 (1972), pp. 671–91.

Stimson, G. V., 'The social background to drug addiction', Proceedings of 5th Symposium on Advanced Medicine, (ed.) R. Williams, Published by Pitman, London (1969), pp. 360–8.

Stimson, G. V., and Ogborne, A., 'Survey of Addicts Prescribed Heroin at London Clinics', *Lancet,* vol. 1 (1970), pp. 1163–6.

Stimson, G. V., and Ogborne, A., 'A survey of a representative sample of addicts prescribed heroin at London clinics', *Bulletin on Narcotics,* vol. 22, no. 4 (1970), pp. 13–22.

Teasdale, J., Segraves, R. T., and Zacune, J., ' "Psychoticism" in drug-users', *British Journal of Social and Clinical Psychology,* vol. 10 (1971), pp. 150–71.

Triesman, D., 'Logical problems in contemporary cannabis and psychedelics research', *International Journal of the Addictions,* vol. 8, no. 4 (1973), pp. 667–82.

Zacune, J., 'A comparison of Canadian narcotic addicts in Great Britain & Canada', *Bulletin on Narcotics,* vol. 23, no. 4 (1971), pp. 41–9.

Zacune, J., and Hensman, C., aided by members of the Addiction Research Unit, *Drugs Alcohol and Tobacco in Britain: The Problems and the Response',* William Heinemann Medical Books (1971).

Zacune, J., Mitcheson, M., and Malone, S., 'Heroin use in a provincial town – one year later', *International Journal of the Addictions,* vol. 4 (1969), pp. 557–70.

Zacune, J., Stimson, G., Ogborne, A., Mitcheson, M., and Kosviner, A., 'The assessment of heroin usage in a provincial community' in H. Steinberg, (ed.), *Scientific Basis of Drug Dependence,* Churchill, London (1969), pp. 323–30.

Index

Abnormal drinking, pointers to 58
Absorption of tobacco smoke 183–91, 192–204
'Abstem' 86
Accommodation and drinking 40, 70
Adamson and Schmale (1965) 98–9
Advertising tobacco 164–5
Agencies for drunkards 144–53: survey 144–5
  case identification 145
  getting co-operation from 146
  knowledge available from 147–8
  Jellinek formula 150–1
Age of drinkers 6, 65, 116
Air pollution from tobacco smoke 183–91
Aitken (1969) 196
Alcoholics and alcoholic agencies 144–53
Alcoholics Anonymous 33, 44, 86, 110;
  self-help from 115–23
Alcoholism Recovery Project 44, 45
Amnesia due to drink 48, 53, 67
Anti-smoking: influences of 180–1;
  suggestions for strategy 165–7
Armstrong (1969) 219
Arrested persons and drink 41–2, 49, 66
Ashton et al. (1970) 193, 202
Astrup (1972) 184, 187
Attendance at Alcoholics Anonymous, frequency of 119, 122
Aversion treatment for drunkards 104–6;
  pilot control 106

Background of 'Skid Row' sample 35
Bahn et al. (1963) 84
Bailey et al. (1962) 136
Ball (1970) 161
Beard and Grandstaff (1970) 187
Berglund (1969) 162
Blom (1967) 97
Bonfiglio and Donadio (1966) 97
Boulding (1967) 215
Bowden and Woodhall (1964) 202
Brandford Hill (1965) 74
Brown, E. 183–91
Brown and Birley (1968) 98–9, 102–3
Bruun (1963) 84
Bynner (1969) 164

Carbon monoxide from tobacco smoke 183–91, 192–204
Cartwright et al. (1960) 163
Cassidy et al. (1957) 98
Central Statistical Office (1971a) 174
Chafetz (1961) 84
Chandler et al. (1971) 55
Characteristics of 'Skid Row' sample 35
Cherns (1967) 211; (1968) 211, 218; (1969) 211; (1970) 212
Chronology of drinking history 88
Cigarettes: prices, and their changes 172–82; absorption from 183–91, 192–204; *see also* Smoking
Cirrhosis rate 74
Classification of court-convicted drunkards (Jellinek's) 68–9
Clinics for treatment of drinkers 93
Coburn et al. (1965) 183
Coefficients, consumption/price in cigarettes 177
Cole, P. V. 183–91, 192–204
Commins and Lawther (1965) 184
Community involvement *see* Alcoholics and alcoholic agencies; Alcoholics Anonymous; Rathcoole experiment; Wives of alcoholics, how they cope
Consumption of cigarettes, pattern changes in 172–82
Cook, Timothy 124–35, 233–7
Cook et al. (1968) 72–3; (1969) 63
Cooper and Maule (1962) 33, 115
Co-operation and Alcoholics Anonymous 116
Court and the drunkard 63–73: demographic data 65–6; symptomatology of dependence 67
Crime and drinking 52–3, 59
Criminal Justice Act, 1967 63, 73, 125
Crude spirit drinking 34, 38

Davies (1962) 56, 97
Davies et al. (1956) 33, 82, 91
Delirium tremens 67
Dependence: on drink and prison 51–6; and the court 67; on smoking 161–2
DHSS (1973) 192, 196

264